Healthcare in Post-Independen

This book analyzes the development of private healthcare in post-Independence Kolkata, India, and the rapid expansion of private nursing homes and hospitals from a historical and sociological perspective. It offers an examination of the changing pattern of the entire healthcare sector, which over recent decades has transformed itself into a profit-making commodity.

The book explores the complexities of the healthcare services in Kolkata with special emphasis on the emergence, growth, role and the changing pattern of private healthcare organizations and the decline or degeneration of the services of public hospitals. Post-1947 India experienced the implementation of new developments in public health services, amongst other vertical programmes, primary health centres, family planning welfare programmes and community health volunteers. Examining the challenges in establishing a comprehensive health service system and the process of market forces in healthcare, the author investigates its linkages with policies of the welfare state.

This book will be of interest to academics in the fields of medical sociology, history of medicine, health and development studies, and South Asian studies.

Amrita Bagchi is Assistant Professor in the Department of History, Bethune College, Kolkata, India.

Routledge Contemporary South Asia Series

For the full list of titles in the series please visit: https://www.routledge.com/
Routledge-Contemporary-South-Asia-Series/book-series/RCSA

Healthcare in Post-Independence India

Kolkata and the Crisis of Private Healthcare Services

Amrita Bagchi

Routledge
Taylor & Francis Group

LONDON AND NEW YORK

First published 2023
by Routledge
4 Park Square, Milton Park, Abingdon, Oxon OX14 4RN

and by Routledge
605 Third Avenue, New York, NY 10158

Routledge is an imprint of the Taylor & Francis Group, an informa business

British Library Cataloguing-in-Publication Data
A catalogue record for this book is available from the British Library

Library of Congress Cataloging-in-Publication Data
A catalog record has been requested for this book

ISBN: 978-0-367-76296-4 (hbk)
ISBN: 978-0-367-77032-7 (pbk)
ISBN: 978-1-003-16947-5 (ebk)

DOI: 10.4324/9781003169475

Typeset in Times New Roman
by Deanta Global Publishing Services, Chennai, India

I dedicate this work to my parents – my ultimate pillar of strength

and

to the memory of all those who have lost their lives due to rampant negligence and corruption in the world of medical care.

Contents

List of Figures and Tables

Preface and Acknowledgement

The structure, development and role of the healthcare sector in post-1947 Kolkata have been for some time an area of academic interest.

Social scientists from all over have been opening up new dimensions on various aspects of the social history of medicine and have looked into the social, economic and political basis of health sector organizations. And the development and growth of the Indian healthcare sector (both private and public) has been widely discussed from various angles. However, I did not find much work on the development of the healthcare sector in Kolkata.

There were essentially three reasons for my zeroing in on Kolkata:

(i)   Doing a similar study for West Bengal as a whole would be immeasurably difficult, if not impossible, for a normal PhD tenure.
(ii) Kolkata, as one of the leading metropolises of independent India, offered a sufficiently rich field for study.
(iii) Being based in Kolkata offered many obvious advantages.

The present book is principally based on my PhD work. In following the developments it became apparent that there was a radical and fascinating change in the pattern and profile of private healthcare in the post-Independence period – from 1947 to the present. And this phenomenon, therefore, was chosen as the subject of inquiry. I have found that it is not only possible to understand and analyze the changes in the nature and scope of private healthcare in Kolkata but that doing so is essential for anyone interested in health history and policy. I, aided by my supervisor, have tried my best. Whether my efforts have really succeeded in illuminating an important aspect of our post-Independence past is for others to decide.

In pursuing my inquiry, I have found help in many quarters. I would like to express my sincerest gratitude to my supervisor Dr Kunal Chattopadhyay, Professor, Department of Comparative Literature (formerly in the Department of History), Jadavpur University, for his guidance and invaluable suggestions and the moral support which had helped me immensely in completing my work. The discussions which I had with him and the inputs which he gave me have been the building blocks of my work.

Words are inadequate to express my obligations to Dr Shantanu Chacraverti, Historian of Science and Environmental Activist, for the continuous guidance and support which he gave me throughout my work. The exchange of ideas with him in every step and also the extremely helpful suggestions rendered by him proved to be pivotal towards the success of my book.

Special mention must be made of Dr Prasanta Ray, Emeritus Professor, Department of Political Science and Department of Sociology, Presidency College, Kolkata, and Honorary Visiting Professor, Institute of Development Studies, Kolkata, for his precious suggestions and his continuous help, which have gone a long way in fine-tuning of this monograph.

I would like to thank Rabindra Nath Bose, Assistant Professor (Retired), Department of Political Science, Presidency College, Kolkata, for his guidance and also for helping me in obtaining valuable data.

I would like to express my heartfelt gratitude to my father-in-law, late Dr Sankar Narayan Chaudhuri, whose continuous guidance, support and precious suggestions have gone a long way in value addition to my book. Although he is no longer with us, I am sure he would have been one of the happiest persons because of the successful completion of my book.

My sincere thanks to late Dr G.P. Shandilya, Medical Practitioner, Kolkata, for his advice and useful insights.

I should acknowledge my debt to Dr Amitabha Chakrabarti, Consultant Cardio-Thoracic Surgeon, Woodlands Hospital and Rabindra Nath Tagore International Institute of Cardiac Sciences. I also wish to thank Shri Siddhartha Sankar Ray, Librarian, Centre for Studies in Social Sciences, Kolkata, for discussing many contemporary issues on health and healthcare. I also desire to express my obligations to Smt Swati Bhattacharya, Assistant Editor, Anandabazar Patrika Private Limited, Prof Anup Roy, Medical Superintendent and Vice-President (MSVP), Calcutta Medical College & Hospital. Ms Banani Ray, Librarian, Departmental Library, Department of History, Jadavpur University, deserves special thanks. I take the opportunity to express my gratitude to late Dr Gouripada Dutta, Chairman, Standing Committee on Health & Family Welfare, West Bengal Legislative Assembly, and to Shri Aloke Kumar Mukherjee, Advisor (HMIS), State & Family Welfare Samity, Department of Health & Family Welfare. Ms Nanda of 'People's for Better Treatment'– an NGO, run by US-based Dr Kunal Saha had immensely helped me collect lots of data on healthcare corruption and abuse. Somdatta Maity, my junior in the Department of History, Jadavpur University, helped me collect the newspaper reports from National Library Archives. I am thankful to Mr Nilanjan Dutta who has helped in copy editing the entire book.

I am grateful to all the staff of Swasthya Bhaban, Kolkata, all the administrators, owners, managers, nurses, attendants, receptionists, health activists and doctors (who were mentioned in my sources) of the nursing homes and private hospitals for responding to the interviews. I am also grateful to the patients and the patient parties of Calcutta Medical College and Hospital for sharing their time in patiently answering my questions.

I am further indebted to the librarians and staff of National Library, Kolkata, Presidency College, Kolkata, Indian Medical Association, Jawaharlal Nehru University, New Delhi, National Institute of Public Finance and Policy, New Delhi, Institute of Development Studies, Kolkata and West Bengal State Legislative Assembly.

I would further like to thank and express my gratitude to those whose names could not be given here due to space constraint though their role has given me enormous support.

Words would be insufficient to express my gratitude to my mother-in-law and husband who have been constant sources of courage and inspiration. I would not have managed to complete my thesis without their support and encouragement. I would also like to thank all my relatives, friends and well-wishers who encouraged me throughout my work and shared the angst and adventure involved in writing this book.

Finally, my ma and baba are the endless sources of motivation throughout my work. They have tolerated my endless grumblings, encouraged me constantly and kept a watchful eye on the progress of the work. They have been with me through it all, and words are inadequate to describe their encouragement and affection. Last but not the least, my twins Shourja Narayan and Sunandini are the constant sources of my impetus in carrying out this laborious task.

Amrita Bagchi

Introduction

In the last five to six decades, several academic works have been undertaken which saw 'health' assuming dimensions wider than the 'physiological'. World Health Organization's definition of health in its constitution clearly demarcates the finer nuances attached to the ideas of health and illness: health now is seen as 'a state of complete physical, mental and social well-being, not merely the absence of disease or infirmity' (the Preamble to the Constitution of WHO as adopted by the International Health Conference, New York, 19 June to 22 July 1946, signed on 22 July 1946 by the representatives of 61 nation states). From the traditional concept in which promoters used to eliminate or alleviate pain, disease and certain social obstacles in order to enable people to live safer and more fulfilled lives, the modern idea of healthcare has undergone considerable ramifications. Healthcare which was earlier being controlled by state authorities is now being dominated by the heterogeneous private sectors dominating around the world. The new approach to health does not go for treating the illness or disease, but rather sustaining the discomfort within the body as this would generate 'profit' which will strengthen the corporatization of the healthcare industry.

Against this backdrop the present book will investigate the development of private healthcare in post-1947 Kolkata from a historical perspective and explore the institutional history of some of the nursing homes and private hospitals. It will tease out the process of the intrusion of the market forces in healthcare and probe its linkages with the policies of the welfare state.

Though the health and healthcare scenario in colonial Bengal has commanded scholarly attention, there was a striking dearth of research on this issue in post-Independence Bengal (West Bengal). And Kolkata (Calcutta), the metropolitan component of the state of West Bengal, has been no exception. Apart from certain official documents, government manuals, newspaper reports and some articles in medical journals, there has been hardly any serious historical effort focusing on the issue of healthcare in post-Independence Kolkata. Yet statistical data on public healthcare exist in government records and documents, although the data fall severely short in terms of quantity, quality and range.

It is with the objective of filling the existing vacuum this book will trace the growth of healthcare institutions in Kolkata during the post-Independence period.

DOI: 10.4324/9781003169475-1

Together with historicizing the roots of the present problems of healthcare services, the book also explores the role of socio-economic and political forces that operate in a certain geographical space and directly influence the character of its healthcare sectors. The 'problems', which the present work proposes, will be studied from a new dimension. It will look into the malpractices and the ethical issues that centre on healthcare services and the medical profession. It will investigate this problem by exploring the complexities of the healthcare services in Kolkata with special emphasis on the emergence, growth, role and the changing pattern of private healthcare services and the decline or degeneration of the services of the public hospitals in the era of neoliberalization.

At the outset, it is however necessary to state that this book intends to study the evolution of the institutionalized private healthcare services (for private healthcare is a broad spectrum that also includes non-institutionalized medicare), i.e., corporate hospitals or tertiary speciality and super speciality private institutions and small private nursing homes providing curative level care, from a historical and sociological perspective. Along with this admission, another aspect needs mentioning, that the emergence of private healthcare and the decline of public hospitals should never be studied in a simplified form of cause-and-effect relationship structure. Both these systems exist in parallel within a certain geographical space, and the emergence of one sector and the decline of another may not be linked in any simple causal relationship. Rather, several other forces operate and influence the rise and fall.

The aim of this work is not merely to trace the increase of the private healthcare sector in Kolkata but to explore the changing pattern of the entire healthcare sector, which has transformed itself into a profit-making industry over the last two decades. Herein, we shall have to look beyond Kolkata; indeed, we will need to place Kolkata in the wider pan-Indian perspective. Exploring the story of the transformation of healthcare in a welfare state is the chief concern of this work. It will examine how a welfare state by undertaking the policy of load shedding invited private capital to invest in healthcare.

Keeping pace with the changes in the global scenario, the healthcare sectors have also undergone a radical transformation. Local and global compulsion in the post-reform period brought about a paradigm shift within the peripheries of the private healthcare sectors.

This research seeks to highlight the changes that mark a break from the old-fashioned nursing homes of a city in a newly independent country to big private hospitals of a 'post-industrial globalized metropolis'. So this study deals with:

- Degenerating public hospitals of Kolkata.
- Displaced small nursing homes.
- Emerging big private (corporate) hospitals.

Against this backdrop, the present volume seeks to pose and try to answer certain questions. They are:

- What was the state of the public healthcare system in Kolkata after 1947? Was it inadequate to meet the need?

- What was the nature of private healthcare in post-1947 Kolkata? Was its development independent or linked with the public sector?
- Is there any paradigmatic shift within the periphery of the private healthcare sector and in the policy documents in the post-liberalization era?
- What are the factors responsible for the growth of private healthcare in Kolkata?
- Why and how did the welfare state accommodate the influx of corporate capital in the health sector?
- How did the transformation of healthcare from a service to a commodity jeopardize common people's access to healthcare?

Though much has been researched on the issues of healthcare in post-Independence India, largely in the cities of Hyderabad and Bombay, no serious efforts were undertaken to deal with the healthcare sector of Kolkata, in the era following Independence. This study will try to fill this gap, although it will essentially confine itself to private healthcare.

Chapter 1, 'Promises and Commitments: The Development of Healthcare Policies and Plans in Independent India', discusses how historically the state in the Indian context from the ancient period looked after the health of its people. With ushering of the colonial period, the British empire introduced the western system of medicine and also formal medical education in India. After Independence, the welfare state promised to provide healthcare to its population. The Bhore Committee Report, the official technical document on public health in newly Independent India, provided the guidelines for the development of health infrastructure. It also recognized the presence and role of private healthcare in India. The chapter discusses the private healthcare sector and privatization of the healthcare services as two entirely different things. There are three phases of the growth of private healthcare in India. It also shows that within the 'promises and the commitments' of the Independent Indian state the interests of the private healthcare sector were also accommodated. Inadequacies of the public resources provided the space for private players in healthcare to flourish.

Chapter 2, 'Changing Paradigm in the Health Sector (Plans, Policies and Reports): Mid-1980s to 2000s', talks of the changes that were accommodated within the policies and reports of the healthcare sector in the post-liberalization phase that also witnessed the gradual retreat of the welfare state and the intrusion of big capital in health services. The World Bank became the prime player in determining the healthcare reforms in developing countries. The chapter also discusses the report of the High-Level Expert Group on the development of Universal Health Coverage that intends to bring about an insurance-based healthcare system strengthening the entry of private capital.

Chapter 3, 'Public Health Sector and the Development of Nursing Homes in an Eastern Indian Metropolis: From Independence to Late 1990s', will focus on the development of public healthcare services (in Section I) and that of nursing homes (in Section II) in Kolkata. Since the post-Independence demographic shift is inextricably linked with the healthcare services, the pattern of population changes, especially the huge in-migration that Kolkata had experienced, posed a direct threat upon healthcare delivery. The growth of private medical establishments (small nursing homes) from the 1940s to the mid-1990s and the recent scenario of private healthcare in the city will be discussed.

Chapter 4, 'Causes behind the Changing Profile of Private Healthcare Sectors', deals with the factors responsible for the development of incremental privatization as well as programmed privatization. The role played by the degenerating public healthcare behind the further development of the private healthcare sector (retreat of the welfare state) will be narrated in this chapter. The neoliberal turn that created the platform for the corporatization of healthcare will be discussed.

Finally, in Chapter 5, 'The Metamorphosis of Private Healthcare', we shall discuss the impact of the structural adjustment programme and the nature of private healthcare in the post-liberalization era. Issues like the reforms of the public hospitals and the subsequent weaknesses and corruptions of private healthcare (impact of the hard selling of healthcare) will also be portrayed.

It is essential to discuss the modes, methods and efforts employed to collect data from various quarters. Since this is an empirical study on contemporary and near-contemporary history, a great deal of emphasis has gone into eliciting information from oral sources. This is also because this was often the only source wherein information was at all available, for government records are pitifully silent on private healthcare. Be it the initial reluctance as well as resistance on the part of the staff of private nursing homes and hospitals or the red-tapism in the government hospitals, this researcher had to face difficulties at every step.

Let us first discuss the scenarios faced in nursing homes and private hospitals. The interviews were arranged either through personal contacts or through establishing contacts through the phone numbers obtained from the list of private healthcare establishments registered under the Clinical Establishment Act. The interviewees consisted primarily of the doctors, administrators, nurses and other staff members of the nursing homes and private hospitals. The initial reaction in almost all the cases was that of resistance and reluctance to help. This may be due to failure on their part to gauge the real purpose of the interviewer. They might have thought that this researcher might have been a medical representative or even a journalist attempting to do a story on the poor conditions of healthcare in West Bengal. The resistance ranged from unwillingness to be interviewed to not divulging proper information on their respective hospitals and nursing homes. In many of the cases, the interviewees showed a tendency to intentionally misrepresent the facts to this researcher. In certain hospitals/nursing homes, the administrators refused to grant an interview, sometimes on the pretext of a shortage of time and sometimes even without citing any plausible reason. It would however be most unfair not to mention the exceptions – that is the few cases where certain doctors and administrators warmly extended their help in providing valuable data and thereby helping in making this research a success. In my opinion, their kind gesture will go a long way in motivating any researcher intending to do research in this particular area.

Now, let us discuss the scenario in the government hospitals. In this section, the focus was on the interviews with the patient and the patient parties. I found these sessions to be more difficult. There were manifold reasons for this. The patient and the patient parties might have been afraid that if they divulged too many details about their first-hand experience, which might not have been too pleasant, they might have to face the flak and wrath of the hospital authorities and not receive proper care and treatment. They might also have been sceptical about my real identity and in all probability thought that I was a journalist intending to do a story on the decaying healthcare system in government hospitals of West Bengal. Another hurdle which I faced in the government hospitals was that I was initially refused entry inside the wards.

To my utter dismay, I noticed that there were many persons loitering inside the wards who were neither members of the hospital staff nor the patient parties and nobody cared about them although they had objections to letting me enter the wards. I was finally permitted to enter the wards after showing the permission letter from the Medical Superintendent and Vice Principal (MSVP), although I could still feel the reluctance.

This section will remain incomplete if I do not mention here two incidents which I went through at Calcutta Medical College. The first incident occurred in the General Medicine Male Ward where I conducted the interview with the patient party while standing beside the corpse of a patient who died eight hours before and was still lying in the adjacent bed. This was itself a prominent manifestation of the sorry state of affairs of the government healthcare system where there was minimal respect for the deceased. A dearth of proper infrastructure indicated that the body of the patient was still lying in the ward eight hours after death. The second incident occurred in the Female Cardiology Ward in the same hospital where a patient showed great enthusiasm in responding to my questionnaire and also supplied me with many valuable data. It seemed that she had looked upon me as some kind of messiah who can bring about a change in her misfortunes. She kept in regular touch with me and also shared many of her personal problems, which, apparently, did not have any connection with my research. In this way, a personal bonding was established with her.

Lastly, it must be mentioned that although the interviews were based on a set of questions framed by me which the interviewee was supposed to respond to, in certain cases it went beyond that and I got access to valuable inputs which exceeded the scope of the questionnaire. This has helped me immensely in my research and thus paved the way for its successful completion.

N.B. 'Calcutta' had been changed to 'Kolkata' in January 2001. In this study 'Kolkata' has been used all through for the sake of uniformity.

1 Promises and Commitments

The Development of Healthcare Policies and Plans in Independent India

Introduction

The welfare state[1] in India, created after Independence, promised to ensure the overall well-being of the people in terms of their physical and mental development. The medical institutions of the twentieth century which India inherited took shape with greater state involvement. The leadership of the Indian National Congress was considerably influenced by the plans and ideas of Fabian socialists and therefore included the state provision of welfare services in their political agenda during the freedom struggle. They emphasized the need to provide free education and healthcare to all citizens.[2] In formulating the plans for social services, they were influenced by the recommendations of the Beveridge Committee Report in providing welfare services.[3] V. Sujatha[4] has pointed out that the influence of and dependence on state agencies and economic arrangements are a crucial part of the health of the population for a nation state's productivity. Three broad phases of Health Sector Development (HSD) can be discerned – first under the British Empire, then in the initial three decades of Independent India and since the end of 1980s a third phase located under the rubric of 'economic globalization'.[5]

But at the same time, private interests and policies towards privatization of healthcare services were accommodated within the model of welfare services. The 'privatization phase' in the Indian scenario is generally traced from the 1980s onwards. A worldwide wave of privatization in every sector during this time led to the influx of private capital in healthcare, too. In the name of "health sector reform", privatization policies and planned privatization programmes made their appearance in the government documents and reports in this period. This move towards planned privatization was due to a global recession, specifically the oil shock of the late 1970s. As a result, there was a tightening of the fiscal constraints on government budget in both developed and developing countries. This period thus witnessed a reduction in public expenditure and a greater role of market in providing healthcare.[6]

But what is striking and important for our study is that in India, both incremental privatization and planned privatization programmes were present prior to this period. Within the promises and commitments of a newly independent welfare

DOI: 10.4324/9781003169475-2

state, there were certain lacunae which provided the platform for the incremental private sector to flourish in an unplanned manner.

Rama V. Baru[7] has argued that in the case of India and several other developing countries, the growth of private hospitals took place during the late 1970s and early 1980s. On the other hand, private healthcare services in their institutionalized forms were present in the early post-Independence era or even in the colonial period. Their emergence should not be studied as a response to the failure of the public sector or as the implementation of programmed privatization which originates from the pro-private government policies.[8]

Thus, what has been put forward by Bennett, McPake and Mills[9] seems more pertinent in respect of our study. Although during the 1970s and early 1980s, the government policy had an almost exclusive focus on the directly provided, publicly funded healthcare, in many instances private providers of one sort or another continued to operate under this policy of relatively benign neglect. Traditional healers and mission hospitals in Sub-Saharan Africa, small clinics operated by private practitioners in much of Asia and some parts of Africa and the ubiquitous private drug sellers existed prior to the current international emphasis on privatization. Particularly in the case of Kolkata, there was a rapid mushrooming of small nursing homes and private clinics (especially maternity homes), which were the outcome of small, independent, private initiatives in the decades of the 1950s, 1960s and 1970s (we will discuss this phenomenon in detail in a subsequent chapter). These private initiatives in the health sector were undoubtedly beyond the ambit of government support or intervention. However, the later conscious attempt to privatize the health sector was indeed the effect of state intervention. Thus, in India, three distinct phases of the emergence of the private healthcare sector can be identified:

(1) The independent initiative of medical practitioners for establishing small private nursing homes and clinics, without the support of the government.

These categories have been termed as 'cottage industry' in healthcare referring to a number individuals or a group of private practitioners offering services that are often organized under a company or group of companies.[10]

(2) The incremental privatization[11] was largely an unplanned response to the failure of the public sector. The development of this phase had a relation to the policies of the welfare state, as there had been a fiscal cutting back on state intervention in the economy and privatizing numerous state-owned enterprises. This move towards private initiatives in healthcare had a link with the world recession of the 1970s, having an adverse impact on the financing of public services that resulted in the growth of markets in the welfare sector.

(3) Programmed privatization[12] originated from the implementation of pro-private government policies. This phase, however, has a wider implication since it marked the corporatization of healthcare services with direct state support. An important development during the 1980s was the influence of multilateral financial institutions like the International Monetary Fund (IMF)

and the World Bank in giving loans to developing countries under the structural adjustment programme for both the economy and the social sectors.[13]

Taking the third point into consideration, we need to point out here that currently the health landscape itself has changed dramatically over the last two decades. The drivers of ill health and the disease burden experienced by countries have become globalized for both infectious and non-communicable diseases such as Ebola, SARS and pandemic influenza, have emerged and conditions endemic to one region have rapidly spread to newer areas. The responses to these pandemics are no longer traditional mandates of nation states. Several multilateral agencies, private American foundations and other non-state actors are playing an increasingly important role in shaping the national policy response to emerging and chronic diseases and in creating new regimes of regulation. This has given rise to a greater role for public–private partnership in global health governance.[14]

Fidler and Calamaras[15] have pointed out that the emergence of the plethora of new actors like hybrid institutions, networks, alliances and frontline groups brought about certain changes in the global health landscape. These unprecedented changes increased the funding for global health and also the salience of global health as 'high politics' or a foreign policy issue became of utmost importance. Even policy implementation, choices of technology and health governance at the country level are now being influenced by these actors. Interestingly, the World Health Organisation, which was the only multilateral agency for the eradication of diseases and providing leadership in global health matters also, transformed its role.

Commercialization in the global health landscape had its implications for policy at the national level. The discourse on new public management served as the premise for the health sector reform (HSR) ideology and the agenda of the 1980s. It privileged markets in restructuring the role of the state and its engagement with public health and healthcare policy.[16]

Along with this phasewise growth of the private healthcare sector, the question of inequalities in accessing health services has also gained momentum in due course.[17] Though globalization has substantially increased health inequalities, even in the early years following Independence, inequalities did exist. The state's commitment to intervene in healthcare was grounded in the Nehruvian development discourse, which posited a government healthcare system in the long run, leading to a progressive reduction in health inequities and ill health. The 1970s and 1980s however witnessed waves of privatization that increased the role of the market and resulted in rising costs and making health inaccessible to a large number of people.[18]

This interface of the role of market forces on the one hand and that of the state on the other characterizes the changing role of healthcare services in the post-reform era. However, the modernist approach to studying global health governance can be well understood if we examine the evolution of state intervention in healthcare.

Role of the State: Historical Evolution

In the past, healers and physicians have been close to monarchs, chieftains and other centres of political power. They were instrumental behind the emergence of dynasties and kingdoms and mediators between the political set-up and the people in many parts of the world like Asia and Africa. The extent of the influence of the state, the pharmaceutical industry and capital investment in hospitals, however, has varied in different parts of the world and undergone multiple transformations over the centuries. Hence, the kind and degree of mutual impact of the state and market on health and medicine depends on the socio-historical experience of the region concerned.[19]

Ancient Period

Archaeological examinations reveal that along with well-planned cities, proper drainage systems and water supply facilities, the public health services in the Indus Valley Civilization were superior to those of any other community of the ancient Orient. Medical knowledge was mostly a combination of religious, magical and empirical rites and procedures.[20]

During the Buddhist period, the state-supported university of Taxila provided medical education to the students. Ashoka founded hospitals all over his empire with medical attendance at state expense. The state also undertook the planting of medicinal herbs and trees and the supply of potable water from wells along the highways. Further evidence of the state's interest in medicine is available from the Chinese pilgrim Hsuan-Tsang.[21]

Medieval Period

Around the twelfth century, the Muslims brought their own physicians with them and thereby introduced a new system of medicine known as 'Unani'.[22] In medieval South India, both state and religious institutions often subsidized and supported medical care.

In 1506, the first hospital was started in Cochin by the Europeans in India for themselves and the Portuguese established the Royal Hospital in 1510. These institutions housed wounded European soldiers giving them proper nutrition and rest.[23] From the seventeenth century onwards early hospitals were opened in Madras (1664), Bombay (1676) and Calcutta (1707–8), manned by European doctors introducing western medicine for treating soldiers.[24]

Historical research on medicine in the seventeenth and eighteenth centuries mentioned that monarchs and chieftains patronized vaids and hakims in the royal court. Providing for the healthcare of pregnant women and infants in the kingdoms seems to have been the prerogative of monarchs and chieftains in the same regions. During the Maratha reign, hospitals were created for the sick, and several welfare measures on health and sanitation were undertaken with the support of the royal treasury.[25]

Thus, the introduction of western medicine especially for soldiers and the practice of indigenous medicine under state patronage from the fifteenth to early years of the eighteenth century went on simultaneously. The British doctors in the hospitals employed Indian assistants who got training in some aspects of modern medicine. In 1740, the Medical Department of East India Company was started with the British military surgeons and Indian assistants, known as native doctors who practised Ayurvedic and Unani treatments and drugs in the early allopathic hospitals.[26]

Colonial Period

In 1764, the East India Company established the Indian Medical Service. European doctors were brought to treat company personnel. However, these doctors were not found so useful for treating certain local diseases. The British personnel often sought help from local healers. Between 1814 and 1835, some processes of mutual involvement between local healers and European medicine took place. An informal training scheme at Calcutta was established on much more substantial grounds in 1822, as a Native Medical Institute (NMI), teaching indigenous and European medicine.[27]

Apart from hegemonization, Mark Harrison mentions that the Europeans' attitude towards Indian systems of medicine underwent a change after 1820. European medical men borrowed extensively from indigenous medicine. They made extensive use of indigenous medical knowledge, using local medicinal plants and consulting Indian medical texts and practitioners of Indian systems of medicine. But the dominance of western medicine was enshrined in the institutions of the colonial state with the abolition of the Native Medical Institute in 1835.[28]

Parallelly, the establishment of three medical colleges in Calcutta, Bombay and Madras in 1835 was an important landmark in the history of health services in the country. These medical colleges followed the guidelines laid down by the General Council of Great Britain. Perhaps no other country outside the western world could match India in this regard.[29]

Conventional histories of medicine are mostly Eurocentric that give a simple, singular and linear account of medicine as if from a primitive past to a glorious present and as happening only in the West. In fact, the health status of the colonized regions was drastically affected by chronic exploitation and the colonial state was not welfare-oriented.[30] Both Ivan Illich and Michael Foucault[31] were also critical of the idea of the steady progress of humankind and argued that every era predisposes society to certain ailments which it then tries to solve. There was cultural assimilation and encounter with the different systems of medicine that posed a challenge to the indigenous system. This initiated several innovations to revive and invigorate native medicine in the light of western medicine. So by no means it was a one-sided or linear process, but rather one of mutual curiosity and learning.[32]

After 1857, the main factors which shaped colonial health policy in India were concerns for the troops and the European civil population. Health was not a priority for the British who by the mid-eighteenth century were ruling large swathes of India's territory. In the late years of the nineteenth century, the colonial government spent 0.15 per cent of their revenues on health compared to 4 per cent spent on education. High death rates of the European troops from 1869 to 1914, over 69 per 1,000, and the impact of malaria, cholera, typhoid and venereal diseases on troops shifted their attention. They also established hospitals in military cantonments and large civil stations that were manned by qualified doctors and nurses as privileged 'enclaves' to exclusively serve their needs.[33]

During this period, hospitals came into being classified into four categories: first, Class I institutions for the army personnel located in cantonments, second, Class II institutions run by municipal bodies for the public, followed by Class III and Class IV institutions run by private parties with or without government help.[34]

The emergence of an organized public health system dates back to the appointment in 1859 of a special Royal Commission to enquire into the cause of the poor physical conditions of the sepoys in the British Indian Army.[35]

D.G. Crawford has mentioned that besides this system of graded hospitals, the British set up temporary lunatic asylums wherever the Europeans resided in sizable numbers. It offered a good business to a few of the surgeons, as initially such mental asylums were put under private management. Some of these asylums were later taken over by the government, and by the 1850s, a few of them were operating in almost every province of British India.

To meet the requirements of chronic and contagious diseases like leprosy, tuberculosis and different kinds of fever, some other sets of hospitals came up from time to time in the form of leper asylums, TB sanatoriums and fever hospitals, respectively.[36]

Along with the establishment of hospitals, sanitary commissioners were appointed in Madras, Bombay and Calcutta between 1863 and 1869 to implement public health measures, establishing the linkage between environmental sanitation and disease. Improvements were noticed in the quality of water, public sanitation and better housing, which reduced morbidity from waterborne diseases like cholera and typhoid from 40 per 1,000 in 1879 to 10 per 1,000 in 1890–1900.[37]

Preventive health measures were accompanied by a series of enactments like the Village Sanitation Act (1889), Contagious Disease Acts (1864 and 1869) and Epidemics Control Act (1897). The vigorous implementation of these acts empowered sanitary officials (particularly in the time of plague) to enter houses, detain, segregate and quarantine those suspected of having the disease, burning down villages rendering over 100,000 people homeless in the process, creating huge resentment among local populations. Local bodies refused to raise revenues through taxation for sanitation and sewerage disposal works and instead accorded a higher priority to the 'cosmetics' of road watering and street lighting. Enforced in the spirit of authoritarian utilitarianism, people responded to these activities with hatred for a foreign power that they perceived to be intruding into their cultural spaces, private beliefs and imposing social ostracism.[38]

Induction of western medicine in India has been one of the components of domination by western civilization. There were two features of this process. First, the military formed the conduit for induction. Second, western medicine was imposed on a pre-existing system of indigenous health practices, which different sections of the society had developed over the millennia. It was almost "automatic that those who played an important role in perpetuating the unjust colonial rule enjoyed the advantage of having access to Western medical services. Reciprocally the exploited masses were kept out".[39]

From 1900 onwards, the popular demand to extend government services was high. Medical practitioners of all kinds came under increasing governmental regulation. The scheme offered a subsidy of Rs 600 per annum for graduates and Rs 400 per annum for licentiates or LMPs (licentiates in medicines were those who qualified in a briefer course in medicine than medical graduates)[40] with a supply of medicine worth Rs 300 per annum if they set up a dispensary in the rural area. The economic depression of 1929 hastened the government's withdrawal from the scheme that came to a standstill after 1931, and no further arrangements for rural medical care were forthcoming.[41]

Meanwhile in 1914, the post of the sanitary commissioner was merged with the post of Director General (DG) of the Indian Medical Service, thereby reducing the importance of public health.[42] Some of India's most eminent medical professionals such as Dr A.R. Ansari, Dr Khan Saheb, Hakim Ajmal Khan, Dr Jeevraj Meheta and Dr N.M. Jaissurya occupied a leadership position in the national struggle. Inspired by the welfare state movements in the United Kingdom and the socialized health services in the Soviet Union, they demanded a more egalitarian health service system and made this demand an important plank in the anticolonial struggle. Dr B.C. Roy at the All India Medical Conference at Lahore in 1929 presented many important facets of health services during the movement.[43]

The rapid growth of the colonial organization for the governance of the country led to the formation of a cadre of medical personnel called the Indian Medical Service (IMS). The IMS had played a key role in the making of health services in the Indian region. In the course of their service in the IMS, the Indian officers were properly socialized and sanitized so that they became 'Brown Englishmen'. Commenting on this aspect in relation to medical education in 1929, B.C. Roy made some pertinent observations on the overwhelming dominance of the IMS in health services. These observations reflect the understandable frustration and anger among those Indian physicians who had acquired high qualifications but were denied access to a large number of posts in the government simply because they did not join the IMS.[44]

The Indian National Congress set up the National Planning Committee (NPC) in 1930. Subhas Chandra Bose, in his capacity as the Congress president, nominated Jawaharlal Nehru as the chairman of the NPC. A sub-committee was established under the chairmanship of Col Santok Singh Sokhey to assess the health scenario and services of the country and recommend measures for improvement. After the submission of its interim report in 1940, a resolution was adopted emphasizing the integration of curative and preventive functions in a single state agency and the responsibility of the state in the maintenance of health conditions.

Another crucial development was the creation of the Indian Medical Council in 1933. It was created after the General Medical Council in Britain expressed concern over the absence of a supervisory authority in India to coordinate the medical courses in various universities. The Indian Medical Council Act of 1933 sought to set up uniform minimum standards of higher medical education and excluded licentiates of allopathy from the all-India register, deeming them unqualified practitioners, though the provincial registers kept their names.[45]

Bhore Committee: Genesis and Impact on the Development of Healthcare Services in Independent India

In 1943, a committee under Joseph Bhore was constituted to examine the state of health in India and to submit a blueprint for action. In 1946, this committee submitted its three-volume *Health Survey and Development Report*. It made certain recommendations based on principles that must guide a health system: being close to the people, provision of care regardless of the ability to pay and the active promotion of positive health through community engagement and linking ill health to environmental hygiene.[46]

The Bhore Committee blueprint drew from the various Health Service Development (HSD) approaches adopted in the first and second worlds. The design for HSD was three-tiered, from primary units to the district hospitals, each modelled as hospitals with additional preventive activities. While the population norm for the number of facilities has been more or less achieved, only a fraction of bed strength and human resources envisaged has been possible (see Table 1.1).[47]

The Report of the Health Survey and Planning Committee[49] (Bhore Committee) portrayed the miserable health conditions of the country on the eve of Independence, as follows:

General death rate	22.4 (per 1,000 population)
Infant mortality rate	162 (per 1,000 live births) maternal
Mortality rate	20 (per 1,000 live births)
Expectation of life at birth	26.45 yrs (females) 26.91 yrs (males)
Death rate of children under 10 yrs	48 per cent
Disease-wise causes of deaths	
Cholera	2.4 per cent
Smallpox	1.1 per cent
Plague	0.5 per cent
Fevers (including malaria)	58.4 per cent
Dysentery	4.2 per cent
Respiratory diseases	7.6 per cent
Others	25.8 per cent

Total	100.0 per cent

All figures are for British India in 1944[50] and do not include the Princely States.

Table 1.1 The Long-Term Programme Personnel[48]

	Medical Officers	Non-Medical Staff	Hospital Beds	Population per Institution
Primary unit	6	78	75 beds	20,000
Secondary unit headquarters	140	358	650	6,00,000
District hospital	239	1,398	2,500	30,00,000

On the eve of Independence, medical services were scattered and highly inadequate, not only in number but also in the kind of medical services they delivered.[51] During this time, British India (population of 300 million) had 17,654 medical graduates, 29,870 licentiates, 7,000 nurses, 750 health visitors, 5,000 midwives, 75 pharmacists and about 1,000 dentists.[52]

The conference of provincial ministers held in October 1946 endorsed the major recommendations of the Bhore Committee but diluted the proposed coverage norms.[53] The committee recommended two types of programmes, long-term and short-term, to improve the health conditions of the country. It emphasized on preventive service and infrastructural networks and recommended to prepare social physicians or 'fully trained' doctors to serve the masses.[54] At that time the country had a doctor population ratio of 1:6300. The committee wanted the ratio to move to 1:2000 and yet recommended the banning of licentiate education and the gradual elimination of this category, which at that time constituted two-thirds of all practising doctors. This created the urgency to enhance the capacities of medical graduate education in the British model rapidly.[55]

It also resolved to make plans for establishing a health centre for every 40,000 people, 30 beds for every five centres and 200 beds in every district; provide safe water to 50 per cent of the population in the next 20 years and 100 per cent in the next 35 years; and ensure adequate sewerage in towns having a population of 50,000 within 10 years.[56]

The conference also accepted the recommendation to merge the two departments of medical services and public health. This meant amalgamating medical treatment for acute care for sick patients along with public health that essentially deals with population or community health such as infectious diseases.[57]

The first Health Ministers' Conference held in 1948 perceived the recommendations of the first Health Policy of Independent India.[58] Following the recommendations of the Committee, primary health centres were constructed in the early 1950s and the first two Five Year Plans followed the recommendations of the Bhore Committee.[59]

Moreover, as the question of financing healthcare was concerned, the committee recommended a fivefold increase in the per-capita outlay from Rs 1.4 to Rs 5.9 with a recurring expenditure of Rs 2.8 per capita for the first five years.[60] In 1946, India was spending 4 per cent of its budget expenditure on health against 20 per cent by the UK and 13 per cent by the US. But the first Health Ministers'

Conference scuttled it, claiming it to be unaffordable. This was not a difficult target to achieve. It would also have been a fruitful investment in people who would contribute to the new economy. Instead, a selective programme-based approach, perhaps under the influence of the American community development model, was opted for and it had become the cornerstone of our development policy in the early years of planning.[61]

This one policy has had a long-lasting negative impact on the shaping of healthcare in the country. While adopting this model, the government rejected the bottoms-up approach recommended by the Indian National Congress' Health Planning Sub-Committee (Sokhey Committee). The chosen policy was in keeping with the Nehruvian internationalist model of modernization, as against the bottoms-up Gandhian vision of development.[62]

The Bhore Committee's standpoint regarding the role of the private practitioners and the private healthcare institutions was, however, confusing. The intrusion of private interests in healthcare, whether in the form of organization or individual practice was not entertained wholeheartedly in the recommendations.

A survey conducted by the Bhore Committee on the medical institutions of pre-Independence India revealed that 27 per cent of allopathic doctors during the 1940s were in government service while the rest were in private practice.[63] The committee report also revealed that 92 per cent of the institutions were maintained from public funds and the remaining were wholly maintained by private agencies.[64]

On the basis of the Committee report, there seemed to be reservations regarding private practice by doctors in government service but as far as the individual private practitioners were concerned, the committee assured them that their interests would not be affected.[65]

The Bhore Committee had strongly recommended a ban on private practice by government doctors. After Independence, this need was felt during the Second Five Year Plan, when the negative impact of private practice on teaching and research in medical colleges came to the surface. However, these recommendations proved difficult to implement. Efforts at banning private practice were short-lived because of the lobbying power of the doctors.[66]

But the recommendations of the Bhore Committee remained unimplemented. The main reason for this and also for the poor performance of other social sectors was the role of the Bombay Plan[67] in shaping India's economic policy. The Bombay Plan directed the nation's economic policy to serve the needs of private capital by making the state invest in heavy industry and economic infrastructure under the cover that such state participation in economic production would foster the evolution of a socialist society. As a result, the welfare sector (health, education, social security and so on) was ignored.[68] Moreover, in the health service sector, the government let the private practice of medicine flourish. For this, the government significantly subsidized the growth of private medical practice by training medical personnel from taxpayer's funds.[69]

Thus, the first policy formulated on health and healthcare in a welfare state like India acknowledged the substantial presence of the private healthcare sector. It also skilfully provided a solid footing for private individual practitioners to flourish. Though the Bhore Committee had championed the role of the state in delivering healthcare, it protected the interests of the private practitioners by assuring that their practices would be safeguarded.

With the medical colleges for the production of doctors getting priority, little attention was paid to the primary and secondary levels of public health service delivery institutions, especially in rural areas. Few jobs were created in the system; therefore, newly minted doctors inevitably went to private practice. Over the years, private doctors became an organized interest lobby that acquired the power to orient policies.[70]

The newly independent countries not only followed broadly the old colonial pattern of health services, which subserved mostly the small elite and urbanized classes, but due to rapid increase in dependence and commercialization of the medical establishment within the ex-colonial countries, these privileged-class-oriented and urban-based health services started to absorb more and more of the national resources. They also developed strong overtones of dependence and commercialization, rapid expansion of the market for the drug industry, both foreign and domestic, more specialization and professionalization and more and more sophisticated medical institutions.[71]

Sujatha Rao[72] has aptly pointed out that what was left behind was a co-opted elite consisting of the western educated, upwardly mobile middle class, which believed that traditional medicine was quackery and allopathy a symbol of modern scientific temper.[73] India's health infrastructure was thus built upon a system of medicine that was contrary to the present-day realities. Thus, the seeds of the conditions that exist today were sown then – a neglected and weak public health policy of a diffident state, fiscal conservatism with low priority and funding for health.[74]

As a victorious power in World War II, Britain with her might and sound system of governance had successfully launched its National Health Scheme in 1947. But India was badly wounded by the world's most massive human migration in western and eastern borders and famine in its eastern states that cost three million lives and inadequate resources available for the development of a well-knit healthcare infrastructure.[75]

Against this backdrop, the newly independent country inherited the modern health services from the British, which was limited in infrastructure. It served the ruling classes and the native gentry comprising only a small portion of the population.

Health Sector Developments (Policies and Infrastructures): 1950s–1980s

After Independence, the health services system of the country was shaped by two political decisions of the new leadership. Following political commitments made during the struggle for Independence, in the Directive Principles of State Policy of the Constitution, the people were made an important plank – particularly for those living in the rural areas.[76]

The other political commitment, which turned out to be of even more importance, was to bring about the desired changes in the health service systems without making any basic changes in the existing machinery of the government.[77]

At the time of Independence, the investment in the health sector was at best marginal. Low levels of spending in the healthcare sector, especially on hospitals, dispensaries, health centres and pharmaceutical production hardly brought about any qualitative change in the health of the population at large.

The first two Five Year Plans followed the Bhore Committee's recommendations, and at the same time the direct influence of the Bombay Plan was reflected. This emphasized not the abolition of private interests but accommodating and in certain spheres even encouraging their growth.

During the First Five Year Plan (1952–1956) emphasis was laid upon meeting the immediate challenges of health problems. Attention was paid to control epidemics and communicable diseases through mass campaigns like (i) provision of water supply and sanitation, (ii) control of malaria, (iii) preventive healthcare of the rural population through health units and mobile units, (iv) health services for mothers and children, (v) education and training and health education, (vi) self-sufficiency in drugs and equipment and (vii) family planning and population control. Emphasis was also given to the construction of hospitals and dispensaries, besides provision for medical education and training, prevention and treatment of venereal diseases, filariasis, tuberculosis, leprosy, cancer and upgradation of mental hospitals (Government of India, 1952). The National Malaria Control Programme was also launched in the same year. The National Water Supply and Sanitation Programme was started in 1954 and the National Filaria Control Programme was commenced in 1955.[78]

Features of the First Five Year Plan[79] are as follows:

- Setting up antenatal and postnatal clinics by NGOs. Licensing of private nursing homes for maternal and child health services.
- The Government of India entered into an agreement with UNICEF and WHO to carry out a countrywide Bacillus Calmette-Guérin (BCG) programme.
- Non-official organizations were encouraged to establish and run tuberculosis treatment institutions and the government was to give them building and maintenance grants provided these institutions were run on a non-profit basis.
- Voluntary organizations were to be stimulated to set up, with state aid, after-care colonies at suitable places in association with tuberculosis treatment institutions. An adequate supply of drugs was to be provided.

During the Second Five Year Plan, emphasis was given to (i) the establishment of institutional facilities to serve as a base from which services could be rendered to the people both locally and in the surrounding areas, (ii) the development of technical manpower through appropriate training programmes and employment of persons trained, (iii) improvement of public health and institutional measures to control communicable diseases, (iv) an active campaign for environmental hygiene and (v) family planning and other supporting programmes for raising the standard of health of the people. International agencies like the WHO and UNICEF also took part in the development of medical and public health schemes in various parts of the country (Government of India, 1956). The Central Health Education Bureau and the Indian Medical Council were established in 1956. The Demographic Research Centres were established in 1957. The Tuberculosis Institute was established in 1959.[80]

India was helped by various international agencies to build the capacity to cope with the situation. Such help resulted in a tendency towards adopting a techno-managerial approach to disease control rather than undertaking the more difficult but sustainable policy of tackling the causative factors and linking disease with social conditions that produce it. Nonetheless dependence on external help also meant a reduced ability to reflect on what is best for us in our context.[81]

During the first two Five Year Plans the basic structural framework of the public healthcare delivery system remained unchanged. Urban areas continued to get over three-fourths of the medical care resources, whereas rural areas received 'special attention' under the Community Development Programme (CDP). History stands in evidence of what this special attention meant. The CDP was failing even before the Second Five Year Plan began. The government's own evaluation reports admitted to this failure.[82]

To evaluate the progress made in the first two plans and to draw up recommendations for the future path of development of health services, the Mudaliar Committee was set up in 1959. The report of the committee recorded that the disease control programmes had some substantial achievements in controlling certain virulent epidemic diseases. Malaria was considered to be under control. Deaths due to malaria, cholera, smallpox, etc. were halved or sharply reduced and the overall morbidity and mortality rates had declined. The death rate had fallen to 21.6 per cent for the period 1956–1961. The expectation of life at birth had risen to 42 years. However, the tuberculosis programme lagged behind. The report also stated that for a million and a half estimated open cases of tuberculosis there were not more than 30,000 beds available.

The Mudaliar Committee further admitted that basic health facilities had not reached at least half the nation. The primary healthcare (PHC) programme was not given the importance it should have been given right from the start. There were only 2,800 PHCs existing by the end of 1961, much less than half the human resources as envisaged by Bhore. Instead of the 'irreducible minimum in staff' recommended by the Bhore Committee, most of the PHCs were understaffed, large numbers of them were being run by auxiliary nurse midwives (ANMs) or public health nurses in charge. The fact was that the doctors were moving into private practice after training at public expense. The emphasis on individual communicable disease programmes was given top priority in the first two plans. But primary health centres through which the gains of the former could be maintained were given only tepid support. The rural areas in the process had very little or no access to them. The condition of the secondary and district hospitals was the same as that of the PHCs.[83] The Mudaliar Committee also estimated the existence of 12,000 hospitals, 185,000 beds and 88,000 doctors in 1961.[84]

The Third Five Year Plan[85] launched in 1961 discussed the problems affecting the provision of PHCs and directed attention to the shortage of health personnel, delays in the construction of PHCs, buildings and staff quarters and inadequate training facilities for the different categories of staff required in the rural areas. While the Third Plan did give serious consideration to the need for more auxiliary personnel, no mention was made of any specific steps to reach this goal. Only lip service was paid to the need for increasing auxiliary personnel but in the actual training and establishment of institutions for these people, inadequate funding became the constant obstacle. On the other hand, the proposed outlays for new medical colleges, the establishment of preventive and social medicine and psychiatric departments and completion of the All India Institute of Medical Sciences and schemes for upgrading departments in medical colleges for postgraduate training and research continued to be high. The urban health structure continued to grow and its sophisticated services and specialities continued to multiply. The Third Plan gave serious consideration to suggesting a realistic solution to the problem of insufficient doctors for rural areas 'that a new short-term course for the training of medical assistants should be instituted and after these assistants had worked for five years at a PHC they could complete their education to become full-fledged doctors and continue in public service'. The Medical Council and the doctors' lobby opposed this and hence it was not taken up seriously.

From the Third Five Year Plan onwards, family planning has remained the main concern of the Ministry of Health. A new Family Planning Department was created in the Ministry of Health in 1966. Since then, nomenclatures may have changed from maternal and child health to child survival and safe motherhood, and presently reproductive and child health under international patronage but the underlying emphasis of the health programme remains family planning or population control. As a consequence, even the poor have to seek primary care from private health providers, often from those not qualified in any system of medicine.[86]

The Second (1956–1961) and Third Plan (1961–1966)[87] pointed to certain key issues:

- Government subsidies and grants were given to states, local authorities, NGOs and scientific institutions for family planning clinics and research relating to demographic issues.
- Maternity and child welfare services provided by the primary health centres were supplemented by services provided by welfare extension projects and by voluntary organizations.
- A large number of voluntary organizations and social workers in anti-leprosy work were to be associated with the leprosy prevention programme.

The Fourth Five Year Plan[88] expressed its concern for the poor progress made in the primary healthcare programme and proposed the construction of speedy construction of buildings and improvement of the performance of PHCs by providing them with staff, equipment and other facilities. For the first time, PHCs were given a separate allocation. It was reiterated that the PHCs' base would be strengthened along with, sub-divisional and district hospitals, which would be referral centres for the PHCs. The importance of PHCs was stressed to consolidate the maintenance phase of the communicable disease programme. In 1966, there had been a steep rise in the incidence of malaria, which rose from 100,000 cases annually between 1963 and 1965 to 149,102. Nutrition, water and sanitation were separated from the Health Department and nutrition came under the Department of Women and Child Development while water and sanitation were attached to the Department of Rural Development.

Family Planning found its place in this plan as a programme of the highest priority. The year 1967 marked the beginning of a steep decline in health services, culminating in the present state of its serious "sickness". An all-out effort to push forward the Family Planning Programme at all costs had a devastating impact on the wider provision of health services. The political leadership permitted bureaucrats to make the people 'targets' of their own 'democratic' government. Owing to the overriding priority given to the Family Planning Programme, plan allocations for it jumped a phenomenal 10,000-fold – from Rs 6.5 million in the First Plan (1950–1955) to Rs 65,000 million in the Eighth Plan (1991–1995).[89]

The Fourth Five Year Plan highlighted that population growth was the central problem and used phrases like 'crippling handicap', 'very serious challenge' and an anti-population growth policy as an 'essential condition of success' to focus the government's attention to accord fertility reduction 'as a program of the highest priority'.

The government acknowledged that despite advances in terms of the infant mortality rate going down and life expectancy going up, the number of medical institutions, functionaries, beds, health facilities, etc. were still inadequate in the rural areas. In the Fifth Five Year Plan,[90] the government accepted that the urban health structure had expanded at the cost of the rural sectors. New methods of family planning, integrated systems for delivery of healthcare services to infants and control and prevention of communicable diseases including malaria, tuberculosis and cholera, besides provision of safe drinking water supply were prioritized in this plan. The concept of family planning was changed into family welfare during this plan period. The country was declared free from smallpox in April 1977. The National Institute of Health and Family Planning was formed and the Rural Health Scheme was launched in 1977.

The Fourth (1969–1974) and Fifth Five Year Plans (1974–1979)[91] emphasized the following issues:

- NGOs to integrate family planning as part of their other health services that they extended to the community, distribution of contraceptives and education.
- In urban areas, it was proposed that private practitioners provide advice, distribute supplies and undertake sterilizations.
- Financial support from the government to private practitioners and NGOs.
- In order to create a sense of partnership with government efforts, voluntary contributions to be encouraged in the malaria programme.

Thus, from the late 1970s onwards, India started to show some positive developments in the vertical programmes that were undertaken in the years following Independence. Some successes were visible in the eradication of smallpox and control of malaria. Overcrowded public and private hospitals were visible in cities and towns. Rural patients had limited access to quality medical care. More emphasis was being given to population control through expanding access to contraceptives. The need for creating the bottoms-up model of the Gandhian vision rather than the Nehruvian internationalist model in healthcare[92] was fully neglected.

Sujatha Rao[93] has pointed out three major developments during the first three decades of India's expansions in health systems.

- Dominant policy focus on family planning and controlling infectious diseases.
- Emphasis on the establishment of teaching hospitals to produce the required human resources.
- Patchy and grossly inadequate funds allocated for the foundation of primary healthcare due to limited weak prioritization and limited resources.

Moreover, several expert committees (more than 25 committees in healthcare) were formed paying little or no significant attention to serious public health issues. Apart from the Mudaliar Committee in 1959, the Chadha Committee (1963), the Mukherjee Committee (1965), the Jungalwalla Committee (1967), the Kartar Singh Committee (1972) and the Srivastava Committee (1975) were set up.[94]

The inadequate attention accorded to the provisioning of medical treatment and hospital care led to the mushrooming of a range of standalone diagnostic clinics, nursing homes and hospitals in the private sector, particularly in urban and semi-urban areas, catering to different socio-economic strata.[95] In the late 1970s, although the public sector provided the most in patient care, there were many signs of strain. There were evidences of poorly equipped and hardly functioning health centres. Ill-motivated staff attended sporadically and treated their poorer patients with barely concealed contempt. Moreover, legally or illegally, many staff members used the public sector to channel their patients into their private consulting practices, or in other ways made use of their public positions for private purposes. Most importantly, the health centre staff preferred to focus on medical care, leaving public health provisions in prevention and care as much as lower priorities, both within the health services and in health planning.[96]

The remarkable achievement through concerted political will of those post-Independence years in controlling diseases has not been sufficiently recognized and applauded in India or abroad. Over the years, though, these programmes lost their momentum and the emphasis shifted from a centralized public sector (that provided preventive and promotive healthcare to all and basic curative services for the poor who could not afford private services) to an uncontrolled private sector that chiefly served the small affluent section with the ability to pay for such services. The indigenous systems of medicine that are cheaper have also been ignored. While 700,000 doctors have been trained in the western allopathic system and an equal number in Ayurveda and homoeopathy, the budgetary allocation for the former is 96 per cent and for the latter, a mere 4 per cent. While as much as 70 per cent of the population is still based in rural areas, 70 per cent of doctors practice in urban areas. This clearly demonstrates the perversity of a political culture that permits a small but affluent section of people to decide policies that favour the affluent few against the poverty-stricken majority. The result is that the 5 per cent of the population in whom the wealth of the country is concentrated is dangerously overmedicalized in five-star hospitals, the middle class is pauperized as it tries to follow its wealthier role model and the poor are forced to rely on an exploitative private sector as the public sector grows increasingly ineffective and unaccountable.[97]

Actually the Indian health sector and health policy makers followed the line of their colonial masters, who believed that germs were the causes of all the diseases and they should be removed from the human body by curative measures. So undertaking long-term preventive measures under the responsibility of the state was overlooked.

The Alma-Ata Declaration of 1978 on primary healthcare, together with the slogan of Health for All by 2000 AD (HFA) proposed at the 1976 World Health Assembly, is considered to be the major public health initiative of the twentieth century. Alma-Ata has since come to be identified with certain basic tenets of public health, such as those of primary health care (PHC), universal access to healthcare and health for all.[98]

Thus, governance architecture for global health has evolved since the International Primary Health Conference in 1978. Led by the World Health Organization, the declaration called upon national and international actors (governments, UN agencies, donors and non-governmental organizations) to support and collaborate in developing and implementing comprehensive primary health care (PHC). It placed special emphasis on the role of nation states in formulating policies and plans to support PHC as part of a comprehensive strategy to build and sustain national health systems and governing matters related to their populations' health. At the heart of this strategy and conception of PHC were communities and their participation in attaining system goals. Since Alma-Ata, the global health landscape started changing significantly.[99]

In India, during this time there was active participation of the civil society and health activists with limited achievements to strengthen the primary-level services through active community participation.

A symposium by the Indian Council for Medical Research (ICMR), held in Hyderabad in late 1976, pulled together accounts of 14 projects, including Jamkhed. The Janata Government of 1977 brought a new set of political actors and provided a new set of avenues of influence. The report of an official committee of social scientists and medical scientists, including Ayurvedic physicians K.N. Udupa and Raremovej Arole, was unofficially published in 1981.[100] These ideas lay behind new schemes for comprehensive primary healthcare in rural areas. A major initiative was launched in 1977, including a massive government programme to recruit – even only for a few weeks – a community health worker (CHW) for each of India's 65,000 villages.[101] All such developments and the recommendations of the Srivastava Committee Report of 1975 resulted in the introduction of the village health worker (VHW) scheme. Under this scheme, every village was to have a VHW who was to provide healthcare services to the community for a small monthly honorarium of Rs 50 and a medical kit. However, this scheme floundered due to the lack of training, supervision and logistic support.[102]

The emphasis on PHC in the Alma-Ata Declaration was an outcome of the failures of the traditional vertical programmes concentrating on specific diseases, as well as of the criticism of the assumption that 'western medical systems' would meet the needs of the common people in developing countries. The 1960s and 1970s was a period of social ferment, of several movements, including the radical science movement in the West. Radical political critiques arose from several quarters, such as from the anti-war movement, from the organized Left and from the women's health movement. There were calls and movements for alternative technologies, for 'appropriate' technology, 'intermediate' technology, as also opposition to ideologies propounding a 'technological imperative'.[103]

The 1981 ICSSR/ICMR[104] report 'Health for All: An Alternative Strategy' offered a viable alternative to this dismal health scenario, especially for the 85 per cent of Indians who were most in need of such services. The report was based on the social, cultural, economic and epidemiological patterns of the vast majority of our people. The aim of this far-sighted report, to which some of the eight most senior members of the medical and social science(s) professions contributed, was to provide an alternative healthcare system that was accessible, culturally acceptable and cost-effective for all citizens, especially the poor, and that was accountable to the people it served. It advocated using the People's Sector as anticipated under Panchayati Raj. Its salient features were:

- Using inherent self-interest, social skills and face-to-face social accountability of the local community.
- Encouraging people to utilize their age-old health culture and practices together with the best of all available systems provided in a simple and effective manner.
- With the support of the community, this decentralized system could devise a graded training and referral system from the village to the community's own hospital and training complex. This would meet almost 95 per cent of all requirements of health and medical care up to a broad-based medical and surgical speciality level within a 30,000-population level presently serviced by the government primary health centres.

The approach bears some resemblance to the 'barefoot doctors' of communist China. This experiment, it is often said, could only have worked in a dictatorial regime like Mao's China. Yet the experience of several NGOs in various parts of India (including Kerala) and other countries has demonstrated similar achievements since the 1970s under democratic, non-dictatorial forms of governance.[105]

Simultaneously during this period, the 34th World Health Assembly was held in Geneva, from 4 to 22 May 1981.[106] The then Prime Minister Mrs Indira Gandhi had participated in the assembly where she had focused on the following issues of the health conditions of the Indian people. She had highlighted that:

> We do need excellent modern hospitals. But the desire for ever larger hospitals, more often than not oriented towards high-cost modern technological medicine, has to be resisted. Primary healthcare must be within reach, in terms of distance as well as money, of all people. The world has found to its dismay that resources are not unlimited. Hence waste of any kind and in any form, particularly in health and hospital care, should be strongly discouraged, and the countries' resources must be more equitably distributed. If this is true of the national scene, it is even more so internationally. In India we should like health to go to homes instead of larger numbers gravitating towards centralized hospitals. Services must begin where people are and where problems arise. We have acquired the capability of placing satellites in orbits which give useful information, but we have not yet been able to reach out to all our rural people. However, we are engaged in reorganizing our medical administration. Our outlook has been admirably expressed in one of the documents prepared by our own doctors, which says, 'Health is neither a commodity to be purchased nor a service to be given; it is a process of knowing, living, participating and being'.
>
> A country's progress is generally judged in terms of its GNP. But surely the health of the people is also a significant yardstick. That is why we must stress the need for a health revolution in developing countries, not only to wipe out diseases and to make available specialized treatment, but what is equally essential, to provide basic healthcare and to take preventive measures. Education from the earliest stages must include certain elementary information about health, sanitation, cleanliness, the avoidance of contagious diseases and the preservation of the environment which is closely linked to these.

The Sixth Plan[107] was to a great extent influenced by the Alma-Ata Declaration of Health For All by 2000 AD and the ICSSR-ICMR report. The plan conceded that

> there is a serious dissatisfaction with the existing model of medical and health services with its emphasis on hospitals, specialisation and super specialisation and highly trained doctors which is availed of mostly by the well to do classes. It is also realised that it is this model which is depriving the rural areas and the poor people of the benefits of good health and medical services.

Key Features of the Sixth Plan (1980–1984)[108] are as follows:

- Encourage private medical professionals and non-governmental agencies for increased investment.
- Government offers organized, logistical, financial and technical support to voluntary agencies active in the health field.
- Encourage the participation of voluntary agencies through financial support in leprosy.
  - Financial assistance to be provided to voluntary organizations which provide medical care facilities at the village level through doctors employed on a part-time basis.

This plan and the Seventh Plan too, like the earlier ones, made a lot of radical statements and recommended progressive measures. But the story was the same – progressive thinking and inadequate action. Whatever new schemes were introduced the core of the existing framework and ideology remained untouched. Privatization was the global characteristic of the 1980s and the 1990s and it made inroads everywhere and especially in the formerly socialist countries.[109]

The Seventh Plan (1985–1990) highlighted the following schemes:[110]

- Voluntary organizations and local bodies encouraged to undertake responsibility for family welfare and primary healthcare services.
- NGOs involved in the extension education and motivation in family planning programme (FPP).
- Scheme for assisting private nursing homes for family planning work continued.
- Increased emphasis laid on Medical College and Hospital (MCH) activities by supporting NGOs, village health committees and women's organizations. Priority assigned to enlist community participation and the aid of voluntary organizations in the leprosy programme.
- Further development of organized blood bank and blood transfusion services with the active participation of the Centre, the states and voluntary organizations.

As a consequence of the debate on alternative strategies during the seventies, the global signing of the Alma-Ata Declaration on Health for All by 2000 AD and the recommendations of the ICMR-ICSSR Joint Panel, the government decided to have a formal health policy. It was felt that an integrated, comprehensive approach towards the future development of medical education and training, research and health services was needed to serve the actual health needs and priorities of the country.[111] After the implementation of the Sixth Five Year Plan (also referred to as the Janata Government Plan, which was revolutionary since it marked a change from the Nehruvian model of Five Year Plans),[112] a demand was raised from all quarters, especially from the health personnel that the Government of India should formulate a National Health Policy (NHP). All the political parties were unanimous regarding the need for an NHP, and a countrywide movement through meetings, seminars and debates was organized to influence the government in formulating the policy. Nevertheless, the Indian Medical Association (IMA) also strongly voiced the need for an NHP.[113] Along with these attempts at the national level, the Alma-Ata conference in 1978 proclaimed that every country should have a declared NHP. Finally, the National Health Policy was formally adopted in parliament in December 1983.

National Health Policy 1983

Though NHP 1983 reiterated some of the progresses achieved in the health sector since Independence, at the same time in the subsection 'The existing picture',[114] the policy highlighted the

> poor health conditions of the people suffering from several communicable and non communicable diseases. Blindness, leprosy and T.B. continue to have a high incidence. Only 31% of the rural population has access to potable water supply and 0.5% enjoys basic sanitation. High incidence of diarrhoeal diseases and other preventable and infectious diseases, especially amongst infants and children, lack of safe drinking water and poor environmental sanitation, poverty and ignorance are among the major contributory causes of the high incidence of disease and mortality.

It criticized the existing situation by describing it as[115]

> largely engendered by the almost wholesale adoption of health manpower development policies and the establishment of curative centres based on the Western models, which are inappropriate and irrelevant to the real needs of our people and the socio-economic conditions obtaining in the country. The hospital-based disease and cure-oriented approach towards the establishment of medical services has provided benefits to the upper crusts of society, especially those residing in the urban areas. The proliferation of this approach has been at the cost of providing comprehensive primary health care services to the entire population, whether residing in the urban or the rural areas. Furthermore, the continued high emphasis on the curative approach has led to the neglect of the preventive, promotive, public health and rehabilitative aspects of health care. The existing approach, instead of improving awareness and building up self-reliance, has tended to enhance dependency and weaken the community's capacity to cope with its problems.

However, the contours of the National Health Policy have to be evolved within a fully integrated planning framework, which seeks to provide universal, comprehensive primary healthcare services; relevant to the actual needs and priorities of the community at a cost which the people can afford, ensuring that the planning and implementation of the various health programmes is through the organized involvement and participation of the community, adequately utilizing the services being rendered by private voluntary organizations active in the health sector.[116]

The salient features of the 1983 health policy were:[117]

a) It was critical of the curative-oriented western model of healthcare.
b) It emphasized a preventive, promotive and rehabilitative PHC approach.
c) It recommended a decentralized system of healthcare, the key features of which were low cost, de-professionalization (use of volunteers and paramedics) and community participation.
d) It called for an expansion of the private curative sector, which would help reduce the government's burden.
e) It recommended the establishment of a nationwide network of epidemiological stations that would facilitate the integration of various health interventions.
f) It set up targets for achievement that were primarily demographic in nature.

As far as the criticism of the NHP 1983 is concerned, three issues should be significantly addressed.[118]

Firstly, have the tasks enlisted in the 1983 NHP been fulfilled as desired?

Secondly, were these tasks and the actions that ensued adequate enough to meet the basic goal of the 1983 NHP of providing 'universal, comprehensive primary healthcare services, relevant to actual needs and priorities of the community'?

Thirdly, did the 1983 NHP sufficiently reflect the ground realities in healthcare provision?

In the decade following 1980, rural healthcare received special attention. Massive infrastructure expansion and programmes for providing primary healthcare facilities were undertaken in the Sixth and Seventh Five Year Plans to achieve the target of one primary health centre (PHC) for 30,000 people and one sub-centre (SC) per 5,000 people in the plains and one PHC for 20,000 people and one sub-centre for 3,000 people in tribal and hilly areas. This target has been more or less achieved in most states.[119] Although the infrastructure is in place in most areas, they are grossly underutilized because of poor facilities, inadequate supplies, insufficient effective person-hours, poor managerial skills of doctors, faulty planning of the mix of health programmes and lack of proper monitoring and evaluatory mechanisms. Furthermore, the system being based on the health team concept failed to work because of the mismatch of training and the work allocated to health workers, inadequate transport facilities, non-availability of appropriate accommodation for the health team and an unbalanced distribution of work time for various activities. Family planning, and more recently immunization, gets a disproportionately large share of the health workers' effective work time.[120]

Among the other tasks listed by the 1983 health policy, decentralization and de-professionalization have taken place in a limited context but there has been no community participation. This is because the model of primary healthcare being implemented in the rural areas has not been acceptable to the people as evidenced by their healthcare-seeking behaviour. The rural population continues to use private care and whenever they use public facilities for primary care it is the urban hospital that they prefer. Let alone provision of primary medical care, the rural healthcare system has not been able to provide for even the epidemiological base that the NHP of 1983 had recommended. Hence, the various national health programmes continue in their earlier disparate forms, as was observed in the NHP.[121]

As regards the demographic and other targets set in the NHP, only the crude death rate and life expectancy have been on schedule. The others, especially fertility and immunization-related targets, are much below expectation. NHP was against 'vertical' programmes and advocated that existing vertical programmes like National Malaria Eradication Programme (NMEP) and Family Welfare (FW) are merged (horizontally) into the healthcare services. In practice, not only was this neglected but new vertical programmes such as AIDS control and separate organizations like the National AIDS Control Organisation were founded outside the Ministry of Health. The National Health Policy advocated an integrated approach. But both multiple health work (MPW) and community health worker (CHW) schemes have been mismanaged to an irrevocable stage.[122]

The National Health Policy of 1983 was in no way an original document. It accepted in principle the ICMR/ICSSR Report (1981) recommendations as is evident from the large number of paragraphs that are common to both documents. But beyond stating the policy, there was no subsequent effort at trying to change the health situation for the better.[123]

The significance of the NHP is enormous with respect to the legitimization of the private healthcare sector in India. This health policy document for the first time mentioned the role of the private sector in delivering healthcare to the population at large. The government made an open reference to the private healthcare sector stating that,

> With a view to reducing Governmental expenditure and fully utilizing untapped resources, the planned programmes may be devised, related to the local requirements and potentials to encourage the establishment of practice by private medical professionals, increased investment by non-governmental agencies establishing curative centres and by offering organized, logistical, financial and technical support to voluntary agencies active in health field.[124]

The NHP is a landmark in the evolution of health services in Independent India because it indicated a shift in the position of the government emphasizing the need for the private health sector.

The government openly declared for the first time that the foundation stone of privatization of healthcare was being laid as an integral part of the state policy.[125]

Meera Chatterjee[126] has analyzed in detail the various aspects of the NHP 1983. The policy statement was the first of its kind, although over the past 40 years, a series of committees had advised the central government on the country's health problems and their solutions. The policy is broad in its approach to health needs and possibilities and ambitious in its goals. Besides acknowledging many mistakes of the past and calling for their redress, it embodies concepts of social justice and democratization, which have been eclipsed in the process of health development.[127]

As far as the question of the private healthcare sector or the privatization process is concerned, Chatterjee argues that the health policy statement makes frequent reference to the need to involve the private medical world (both individual practitioners and voluntary agencies) closely with the government health efforts. However, the policy does not specify how the government will coordinate with the private sector. The goal of 'health for all' can be a 'collective responsibility' only if the actions of each partner are clearly defined and well-coordinated.[128]

The policy statement suggests that the services being rendered by the private and voluntary health agencies should be adequately 'utilized' by the government in the provision of universal primary healthcare. In addition, the government is to encourage new voluntary efforts in the cause of health for rural and urban slum areas. It is envisioned that voluntary agencies' 'service and support would require to be utilised and intermeshed with the governmental efforts, in an integrated manner'. Analogously, the services of private indigenous practitioners are also to be 'integrated' into the overall health delivery system for 'preventive, promotive and public health objectives', but those of private allopathic practitioners have been excluded from this intention.[129]

The policy also mentioned that along with joining hands with the private healthcare sector for primary healthcare, the government also wished to increase investment by private agencies in curative medical centres, particularly 'speciality' and 'super-speciality' facilities, to ensure that they were adequately available within the country. Chatterjee rightly argues that the avowed intention here is to reduce government spending on these so that more money becomes available for basic health services and existing government curative facilities are eventually used to treat the needy. To achieve this, it is proposed that the government offer logistic, financial and technical support to the private medical sector.[130]

Thus, in the spirit of 'privatization', the government is devolving on the private sector some responsibilities. If the health sector is viewed as a conventional pyramidal structure, government services would be limited to the intermediate levels, while private agencies occupy the bottom of the pyramid. Their situation implies that both community-based voluntary agencies and sophisticated urban medical organizations will have 'interfaces' with the government health system.[131]

However, the NHP 1983 has been strongly criticized by several sections for its pro-private orientation. One of the senior physicians of Kolkata thinks that perhaps the saddest part of the whole health policy statement lies in inviting private agencies to replace the government efforts. According to him, the government in no circumstances can abdicate its final responsibility of ensuring people's health nor can it allow private profit seekers to flourish at the expense of people's welfare.[132]

Chatterjee has pointed out certain possibilities for justifying the government's pro-private approach towards the healthcare sector.[133] These are:

- In a fundamental way, privatization signifies the government's desire to expand private enterprise in all spheres of health in order to increase people's access to healthcare. By the absorption of private agencies and personnel in state policy and programmes the 'joint' health sector may receive a fillip so that it becomes bigger, more varied and more effective.
- At this juncture 'privatization' may be a part of a strategy for decentralization, necessary to achieve better results in health, just as in other development sectors such as agriculture and education. This may help to circumvent a major problem encountered in governmental efforts to decentralize.
- The desire of the government to privatize means involving voluntary agencies in national health development to meet policy and planning objectives and targets. The decentralized and socially committed nature of the voluntary sector and its superior ability to organize people compared with bureaucratic structures are given as reasons for privatization.
- It has been further argued that privatization is a strategy to co-opt the voluntary sector in order to quell shouts about bureaucratic inefficiency, corruption and so on and to dilute threats to the existing power structure. In this view, the provision of funds or technical assistance to voluntary agencies, the placement of private sector leaders in governmental committees or giving consultancies to them are considered tactics of diffusion.
- Finally, privatization has been identified with the process of 'de-nationalization'. Although devolution may be gradual, the government may hope eventually to turn over the provision of healthcare entirely to the private sector. This aspiration may stem from the realization that despite the immense resources the state has sunk into health services over the years, it still fails to reach the majority of the people. The corollary of de-nationalization is greater privatization of the state, which is increasing reservation of government health services for 'the few'.

Thus, India, being a welfare state, had not only provided deliberate space for the private healthcare sector to flourish but at the same time, it has given legitimization to this sector by mentioning its considerable role in health services. The government took proficient measures to establish the private healthcare sector in India as the remedy against the degenerating condition of public healthcare, which was the result of their intentional act of shirking their basic responsibilities. The promotion of a capitalist economy in every sector resulted in transforming healthcare from a service to a commodity and the state took deliberate but subtle steps for fostering this development.

NHP did not bring about any basic change in the 'architecture' of the health system: the budget for health continued to be low and the approach to adopting selective healthcare delivery remained the same.[134]

From the above discussion it is thus clear that prior to the advent of the process of economic globalization in India, the private healthcare sector not only occupied a considerable physical space but also made its appearance in the policy documents. So, the conventional way of identifying the 'prescription' behind the emergence of the private healthcare sector in India along with other developing countries with the publication of the World Development Report 1993 subtitled Investing in Health Care cannot be fully accepted.

Between Independence and till mid-1980s, the growth of the state health sector has not kept pace with the needs of the population. On the other hand, the private health sector has grown from strength to strength because there is a vast demand which must be met. The government has failed to meet this demand but the private sector has served it, in whatever manner or quality.[135]

The Seventh Five Year Plan accepted the above NHP advice. It recommended that 'development of specialities and super-specialities need to be pursued with proper attention to regional distribution' and such 'development of specialisation and training in super-specialities would be encouraged in the public and the private sectors'. This plan also talks of improvement and further support for urban health services, biotechnology and medical electronics and non-communicable diseases. Enhanced support for population control activities also continues. The special attention that AIDS, cancer and coronary heart diseases are receiving and the current boom of the diagnostic industry and corporate hospitals are a clear indication of where the health sector priorities lie.[136]

It took India almost 35 years of Independence before announcing its first National Health Policy in 1983. The phenomenon of rising public investment in health was, however, short-lived. It began in the early 1980s and ended even before the start of the 1990s, the liberalization phase in the Indian economy.[137]

Tectonic shifts were taking place on the global stage. By the late 1970s and early 1980s, socialism was beginning to lose its influence on market forces. The concept of a welfare state that had emerged at the end of World War II in post-war Britain was being replaced and redefined by the state as a facilitator and financier of private enterprise. The post-war prosperity gave rise to new thinking: solidarity gave way to individualism and state to markets. In the 1960s, economists in the US began to argue that health was as much a marketable commodity as any other, making way for markets in the health sector. Led by Ronald Reagan in the US and Margaret Thatcher in the UK, this ideological shift began to impact thinking in India. This resulted in the deteriorating economic environment and the shift towards the liberalization of the economy affecting the healthcare sector in India.[138]

Notes

1 G. Borker, *Health in Independent India* (New Delhi: Ministry of Health and Family Welfare, 1960), 3.

According to Borker, the 'Little Man' had at last come into his own. For one thing, he was the master in his own house, governed by people of his choice as his representatives and responsible to him. Politically, economically and socially he was well on the way to complete emancipation. He had no longer to look to the

'*Ma-BaapSarkar*' (paternalistic government) for scraps but could demand, as a right, all that an individual requires, not merely for existence, but to live as a free and complete human being. To affect this, just a change in government was not enough, but a change of heart was needed.

2   Rama V. Baru, *Private Health Care in India: Social Characteristics and Trends* (New Delhi: Sage Publications, 1998), 46 (hereafter cited as Baru, *Private Health Care in India*).

3   For details of the Beveridge Plan see Michael Foucault, "The Crisis of Medicine or the Crisis of Antimedicine?" translated by Edgar C. Knowlton Jr., William J. Kingand and Clare O'Farrell, *Foucault Studies* 1 (2004): 5–19.

4   V. Sujatha, *Sociology of Health and Medicine: New Perspectives* (New Delhi: OUP, 2014), xiv, 143. (Hereafter cited as Sujatha, *Sociology of Health and Medicine: New Perspectives).*

5   Ritu Priya, "State, Community, and Primary Health Care: Empowering or Disempowering Discourses?", in *Equity and Access: Health Care Studies in India*, ed. Purendra Prasad and Amar Jessani (New Delhi: OUP, 2018), 28.

6   See Sarah Hodges and Mohan Rao, *Public Health and Private Wealth: Stem Cells, Surrogates and Other Strategic Bodies* (Delhi: Oxford University Press, 2016); Purnendra N. Prasad, "State, Community Health Insurance and Commodification of Health Care: A Case of Arogyasri in Andhra Pradesh", in *Medical Insurance Schemes for the Poor — Who Benefits*, ed. Rama V. Baru (New Delhi: Academic Foundation, 2015); Rama V. Baru et al., "Inequities to Access Health Services in India: Caste, Class, Region", *Economic and Political Weekly* 45, no. 38 (2010): 49–58.

7   Baru, *Private Health Care in India*, 40.

8   Sara Bennet, Barbara McPake, and Anne Mills, "The Public/Private Mix Debate in Health Care", in *Private Health Providers in Developing Countries – Serving the Public Interest?*, ed. Sara Bennet, Barbara McPake, and Anne Mills (London: Zed Books, 1997), 5. (Hereafter cited as Bennet, McPake, and Mills, "The Public/Private Mix Debate in Health Care").

9   Ibid., 3.

10 Rama V. Baru and Anuj Kapilashrami, "Unpackaging the Private Sector in Health Policy and Services", in *Global Health Governance and Commercialisation of Public Health in India: Actors, Institutions and Dialectics of Global and Local*, ed. Anuj Kapilashrami and Rama V. Baru (London: Routledge, 2019), 116. (Hereafter cited as Kapilashrami and Baru, "Unpackaging the Private Sector").

11 Bennet, McPake, and Mills, "The Public/Private Mix Debate in Health Care", 5.

12 Ibid., 5.

13 Rama V. Baru, "Health Sector Reform: The Indian Experience", in *Health Care Reform around the World*, ed. Andrew C. Twaddle (Connecticut: Auburn House, 2002), 268.

14 Anuj Kapilashrami and Rama V. Baru, "Global Health Governance and Commercialisation of Public Health in India: Actors, Institutions and Dialectics of Global and Local", in *Global Health Governance and Commercialisation of Public Health in India: Actors, Institutions and Dialectics of Global and Local*, ed. Anuj Kapilashrami and Rama V. Baru (UK: Routledge, 2019), 1–2 (hereafter cited as Kapilashrami and Baru, *Global Health Governance and Commercialisation*).

15 D.P. Fidler and J.L. Calamaras, "*The Challenges of Global Health Governance,*" Council on Foreign Relations, New York, Incorporated. Working Chapter, cited in Kapilashrami and Baru, *Global Health Governance and Commercialisation*, 2.

16 Ibid., 3.

17 Purnendra Prasad, "Introduction: Health Inequities in India — The Larger Dimensions", in *Equity and Access: Health Care Studies in India*, ed. Purnendra Prasad and Amar Jesani (New Delhi: India, 2018), 2–3.

18 Ibid., 2.

19 Sujatha, *Sociology of Health and Medicine: New Perspectives*, 142–43.
20 Henry E. Sigerist, *A History of Medicine: Early Greek, Hindu and Persian Medicine* (New York: OUP, 1961), Vol. 2, 141–42.
21 D.D. Kosambi, *An Introduction to the Study of Indian History* (Bombay: Popular Prakashan, 1975), revised 2nd edition; Romila Thapar, *The Penguin History of Early India: From Origins to AD 1300* (New Delhi: Penguin, 2002); Romila Thapar, *Ashoka and the Decline of the Mauryas* (Oxford: OUP, 1973).
22 Seema Alavi, "Unani Medicine in the Nineteenth-Century Public Sphere: Urdu Texts and Oudh Akbar", *Indian Economic and Social History Review* 42 (March 2005): 101–29.
23 M.N. Pearson, "The Portuguese State and the Medicine in Sixteenth Century Goa", in *The Portuguese and the Socio Cultural Changes in India, 1500–1800*, ed. K.S. Mathew, Teotonio R. de Souza, and Pius Malekandathil, 401–19 (Panaji: Fundacao Oriente, 2001), cited in Sujatha, *Sociology of Health and Medicine: New Perspectives*, 154.
24 Aneeta Minocha, "Women in Modern Medicine and Indian Tradition", in *Social Structure and Change: Women in Indian Society*, Vol. 2, ed. A.M. Shah, B.S. Baviskar, and E.A. Ramaswamy, 150–78 (New Delhi: Sage Publications, 1996), cited in Sujatha, *Sociology of Health and Medicine: New Perspectives*, 154.
25 For details see C.A. Bayley, *Empire and Information: Intelligence Gathering and Social Communication in India, 1780–1870* (Cambridge: Cambridge University Press, 1996); K.R. Krishnan, "Siddha Medicine during the Period of Marattias", in *Heritage of the Tamils: Siddha Medicine*, edited by S.V. Subramanian and V.R. Madhavan (Madras: International Institute of Tamil Studies, 1983).
26 Aneeta Minocha, "Women in Modern Medicine and Indian Tradition", in *Social Structure and Change: Women in Indian Society*, Vol. 2, ed. A.M. Shah, B.S. Baviskar, and E.A. Ramaswamy, 150–78 (New Delhi: Sage Publications, 1996), cited in Sujatha, *Sociology of Health and Medicine: New Perspectives*, 154.
27 Roger Jeffrey, *Politics of Health in India* (CA: University of California Press, 1988), 51. For the details of Native Medical Institute see Poonam Bala, *Imperialism and Medicine in Bengal: A Socio-Historical Perspective* (Sage Publications, 1991); Samita Sen and Anirban Das, "A History of the Calcutta Medical College and Hospital, 1835–1936", in *History of Science, Philosophy and Culture in Indian Civilization*, xv; Uma Dasgupta, ed. *Science and Modern India: An Institutional History, c 1784–c 1947* (Delhi: Centre for Studies in Civilizations, 2011).
28 Biswamaoy Pati and Mark Harrison, *Health Medicine and Empire Perspectives on Colonial Medicine* (New Delhi: OUP, 2001), 37–87.
29 D.G. Crawford, "Notes on the Early Hospitals of Calcutta", *Indian Medical Gazette* 38, no. 1 (1903).
30 Sujatha, *Sociology of Health and Medicine: New Perspectives*, 144. Also see Kapil Raj, *Relocating Modern Science: Circulation and Construction of Scientific Knowledge in South Asia and Europe* (Delhi: Permanent Black, 2006).
31 V. Sujatha in her *Sociology of Health and Medicine: New Perspectives* (Chapter 4: Health, Medicine and State) has cited the arguments put forward by Ivan Illich in his *Medical Nemesis: The Expropriation of Health* (New York: Pantheon Books, 1976) and Michel Foucault in his *The Birth of the Clinic: An Archaeology of Medical Perception* (New York: Vintage Books, 1975). For the study of hegemonization of western medicine and the counter argument on the development of a medical interaction and exchange leading to growth of a shared medical knowledge, which operated outside the dynamics of state power, created a cultural space, where plural notions of disease, body and therapeutics circulated, see David Arnold, *Colonizing the Body: State Medicine and Epidemic Disease in Nineteenth Century India* (Berkeley: University of California Press, 1993); Roy Porter, *Health for Sale: Quackery in England, 1660–185* (Manchester: Manchester University Press, 1989); Projit Bihari

Mukharji, *Nationalizing the Body: The Medical Market, Print and Daktari Medicine* (New York: Anthem Press, 2009); Madhuri Sharma, *Indigenous and Western Medicine in Colonial India, Culture and Environment in South Asia* (New Delhi: Foundation Books, 2012) and Rachel Berger, *Ayurveda Made Modern: Political Histories of Indigenous Medicine in North India, 1900–1955*, Cambridge Imperial and Post-colonial Studies Series (New York: Palgrave Macmillan, 2013); Ratnabir Guha, "Native Bodies, Medical Market and 'Conflicting' Medical 'Systems': Venereal Diseases and the 'Vernacularisation' of Western Medical Knowledge in Colonial Bengal", *Presidency Historical Review* 1, no. 1 (March 13, 2015): 11–18.

32 Sujatha, *Sociology of Health and Medicine: New Perspectives*, 146.

33 K. Sujatha Rao, *Do We Care? India's Health System* (New Delhi: OUP, 2020), 8. (Hereafter cited as Rao, *Do We Care?*) Also see Debabar Bannerji, "Landmarks in the Development of Health Services in India", in *Public Health and Poverty of Reform*, ed. Imrana Qadeer, Kasturi Sen and. K.R. Nayar (New Delhi: Sage Publications, 2001), 41 (hereafter cited as Bannerji, "Landmarks in the Development of Health Services in India").

34 Sujatha, *Sociology of Health and Medicine: New Perspectives*, 155. Also see D.M. Muir, "Notes on the Origin of the Presidency General Hospital Calcutta", *Indian Medical Gazzette* 38, no. 1 (1903); Anil Kumar, "Emergence of Western Medical Institutions in India, 1822–1911" (hereafter cited as Kumar, "Emergence of Western Medical Institutions in India") in *History of Medicine in India: The Medical Encounter*, ed. Chittyabrata Palit and Achintya Dutta (Delhi: Kalpaaz Publication, 2005).

35 K.N. Rao, "Public Health and Health Services", *Encyclopaedia of Social Work*, Vol. I (New Delhi: Publication Division, 1995), 364.

36 For details in the development of hospitals see Kumar, *Emergence of Western Medical Institutions in India*.

37 Rao, *Do We Care?*, 8.

38 Ibid., 8–9.

39 Bannerji, "Landmarks in the Development of Health Services in India", 41.

40 Sujatha, *Sociology of Medicine*, 161.

41 Ibid., 161.

42 Rao, *Do We Care?*, 9.

43 B.C. Roy, "The Future of Medical Profession in India", Reprint of the Presidential Address delivered at the All India Medical Conference at Lahore in 1929, *Journal of Indian Medical Association*, 78 (1 and 2) (1982): 24–30, referred in Banerji, *Landmarks in the Development of Health Services*, 43.

44 Ibid., 41.

45 Sujatha, *Sociology of Medicine*, 162.

46 Rao, *Do We Care?*, 9.

47 Priya, "State, Community, and Primary Health Care", 29.

48 Government of India, *Health Survey and Development Committee (Bhore Committee) Report*, Vol. 2.

49 Government of India, *Health Survey and Development Committee (Bhore Committee) Report*, Vol. 1–4 (New Delhi: Manager of Publications, 1946).

50 When the Bhore Committee set out to examine the state of the health sector in India it had only one estimate of private household expenditure. This was R.B. Lal's Singur study which showed that in 1944 private household expenditure on healthcare was Rs 2½ per capita. In comparison the state health expenditure in the same year was only 36 paise per capita. This totalled up to 4 per cent of the GDP with private health expenditure having a share of 87 per cent.

51 Banerji, "Landmarks in the Development of Health Services", 42.

52 Government of India, *Health Survey and Development Committee (Bhore Committee) Report*, Vol. 1.

53 Minutes of the meetings available with the National Archives of India, New Delhi, referred in Rao, *Do We Care?*, 9.
54 Government of India, *Health Survey and Development Committee (Bhore Committee) Report*, Vol. II, 17–32.
55 Priya, "State, Community, and Primary Health Care", 29. Also see Rao, *Do We Care?*, 9.
56 Rao, *Do We Care?*, 9–10.
57 Ibid., 9–10.
58 Alok Mukhopadhyay, ed. *Report of the Independent Commission on Health in India* (New Delhi: Voluntary Health Associations of India, 1997), 35 (Hereafter cited as Mukhopadhyay, *Report of the Independent Commission*).
59 Meera Chatterjee, *Implementing Health Policy* (New Delhi: Manohar, 1988), 7.
60 GOI, *1946: Health Survey and Development Committee Report*, Vol. II, 510.
61 Ravi Duggal, Where Are We Today?, *Seminar Web Edition*, Monthly Symposium, New Delhi.
62 Ritu Priya, "Public Health Services in India: A Historical Perspective", in *Review of Healthcare in India*, ed. L.V. Gangolli, R. Duggal, and A. Shukla, 41–74 (Mumbai: Centre for Enquiry into Health and Allied Themes), cited in Priya, "State, Community, and Primary Health Care", 30.
63 Government of India, *Report on the Health Survey and Development Committee (Bhore Committee)*, Vol. 1, 1946, 42–43.
64 Ibid., p. 13.
65 Baru, *Private Health Care in India*, 49.
66 Baru, *Private Health Care in India*, 49.
67 For details of Bombay Plan see P. Thakurdas et al., *Brief Memorandum Outlining a Plan of Economic Development for India* (Bombay Plan) (London: Penguin Books, 1946).
68 Ravi Duggal and N.H. Antia, "Health Financing in India: A Review and an Agenda", in *Paying for India's Health Care*, ed. Peter Berman and M.E. Khan (New Delhi: Sage Publications, 1993), 54–55.
69 Ravi Duggal, "Medical Education in India: Who Pays?", *Radical Journal of Health* 3, no. 4 (March 1989). (Hereafter cited as Duggal, "Medical Education in India") Also see Ravi Duggal, "Historical Review of Health Policy Making", in *Review of Healthcare in India*, ed. Leena V. Gangolli, Ravi Duggal, and Abhay Shukla (Centre for Enquiry into Health and Allied Themes, 2005), 28. (Hereafter cited as Duggal, "Historical Review of Health Policy Making").
70 Priya, "State, Community, and Primary Health Care", 30.
71 Debabar Banerji, "Political Dimensions of Health and Health Services", *Economic and Political Weekly*, Vol. XIII, no. 22 (1978): 926. Also see Mukhopadhyay, *Report of the Independent Commission*. Priya, "State, Community, and Primary Health Care".
72 Rao, *Do We Care?*, 10–11.
73 See David Hardiman and Projit Behari Mukherjee, *Medical Marginality in South Asia: Situating Subaltern Therapeutics* (London and New York: Routledge) cited in Priya, "State, Community, and Primary Health Care".
74 Rao, op. cit., 10–11.
75 Ibid.
76 D.D. Basu, *Shorter Constitution of India* (Calcutta: S.C. Sarkar, 1981), 230–35.
77 Ibid., 3.
78 Government of India, *The First Five Year Plan* (New Delhi: Planning Commission, 1952).
79 Rama V. Baru and Madhurima Nundy, "Blurring of Boundaries: Public-Private Partnerships in Health Services in India", *Economic and Political Weekly* 43, no. 4

(January–February 2008): 62–63. (Hereafter cited as Baru and Nundy, "Blurring of Boundaries").

80 Government of India, *The Second Five Year Plan* (Planning Commission, 1956).
81 Rao, *Do We Care?*, 12.
82 Duggal, "Historical Review of Health Policy Making", 28. Also see Priya, State, Community, and Primary Health Care, 34.
83 Mudaliar Committee, 1961: *Health Survey and Planning Committee*, MoHFW, New Delhi.
84 Ibid.
85 Government of India (1960) Third Five-Year Plan: A draft outline, Planning Commission, New Delhi in http://planningcommission.nic.in/plans/planrel/fiveyr/welcome.html, accessed on 30.10.2021.
86 Ibid. Also see Ravi Duggal, Where are we Today?, *Seminar Web Edition, Monthly Symposium*, New Delhi.
87 Baru and Nundy, Blurring of Boundaries, 63.
88 Planning Commission, Government of India, *Fourth Five Year Plan*. New Delhi: Planning Commission, Government of India, 1969.
89 Debabar Bannerji, 'Landmarks in the Development of Health Services in India', 46. Also ImranaQadeer,' Continuities and Discontinuities in Public Health: Indian Experience', in *Maladies, Preventives and Curatives: Debates in Public Health Care*, ed. Amiya Bagchi and Krishna Soman, (Kolkata: Tulika Books, 2005), 88.
90 Government of India (1975) *Draft Fifth Five Year Plan*, Planning Commission, New Delhi.
91 Baru and Nundy, "Blurring of Boundaries",63.
92 For details see Ritu Priya, "Public Health Services in India: A Historical Perspective" In *Review of Healthcare in India*, L.V. Gangolli, R. Duggal and A. Shukla (eds) pp. 41–74, Mumbai: Centre for Enquiry into Health and Allied Themes, Roger Jeffrey, "Medical education: Sound and fury signifying nothing", *Economic and Political Weekly*, 11(1), (1976), 92-93.
93 Rao, *Do We Care?*, 13. Also see Bannerji, 'Landmarks in the Development of Health services in India'.
94 For details of the Committee Reports see http://nhp.gov.in/health-policies_pg. Also see Duggal, "Historical Review of Health Policy Making".
95 Rao, *Do We Care?*, 13.
96 Roger Jeffery, "Commercialisation in Health Service", in *Global Health Governance and Commercialisation of Public Health in India: Actors, Institutions and Dialectics of Global and Local*, ed. Anuj Kapilashrami and Rama V. Baru (UK: Routledge, 2019), 78–79.
97 Noshir Antia Seerna Deodhar Nerges Mistry, *Developing an Alternative Strategy for Achieving Health for All The ICSSR/ICMR Model – The FRCH Experience* (Pune: The Foundation for Research in Community Health, 2004), 7–8.
98 See *Declaration of Alma-Ata International Conference on Primary Health Care*, Alma-Ata, USSR, 6–12 September 1978. Also see Indira Chakravarthy, "Role of World Health Organisation", *Economic and Political Weekly* 43, no. 47 (2008): 41–46. (Hereafter cited as Chakravarthy, "Role of World Health Organisation").
99 Anuj Kapilashrami, "Mapping the Conceptual Terrain of Global Health Governance", in *Global Health Governance and Commercialisation of Public Health in India: Actors, Institutions and Dialectics of Global and Local*, ed. Anuj Kapilashrami and Rama V. Baru (UK: Routledge, 2019), 16.
100 Ramalingaswamy et al., *Health for All: An Alternative Strategy* (Pune: Indian Institute for Education, 1981) cited in Roger Jeffrey, "Commercialisation in Health Service", in *Global Health Governance and Commercialisation of Public Health in India: Actors, Institutions and Dialectics of Global and Local*, ed. Anuj Kapilashrami and Rama V. Baru (UK: Routledge, 2019), 78–79.

101 Charles Leslie, "What Caused India's Massive Community Health Workers Scheme: A Sociology of Knowledge", *Social Science and Medicine* 21, no. 8 (1985): 923–39 cited in Roger Jeffrey, "Commercialisation in Health Service", in *Global Health Governance and Commercialisation of Public Health in India: Actors, Institutions and Dialectics of Global and Local*, ed. Anuj Kapilashrami and Rama V. Baru (UK: Routledge, 2019), 78–79.
102 Rao, *Do We Care?*, 14.
103 Chakravarthy, "Role of World Health Organisation", 41.
104 ICSSR/ICMR (1981): *Health for All: An Alternative Strategy*, Indian Institute of Education, Pune.
105 Ibid.
106 World Health Organisation, *Thirty-Fourth World Health Assembly*, Geneva, 4–22 May 1981. *Verbatim Records of Plenary Meetings and Reports of Committees.*
107 Planning Commission, Government of India, *Sixth Five Year Plan 1980–85* (New Delhi: Planning Commission, Government of India, 1985).
108 Baru and Nundy, "Blurring of Boundaries", 63.
109 Duggal, "Historical Review of Health Policy Making", 33.
110 Baru and Nundy, "Blurring of Boundaries", 63.
111 Mukhopadhyay, *Report of the Independent Commission*, 36–37.
112 Sathia Suthanthiraveeran, *The Five Years Plans in India, Overview of Public Health Policies*, https://www.researchgate.net/publication/327238255, accessed on 08.11.2021.
113 Biswanath Paria, *An Appeal* (Kolkata: Medical Service Centre, 1985), 9 (Hereafter cited as Paria, *An Appeal*).
114 MoHFW, *National Health Policy* (New Delhi: Govt. of India, Ministry of Health & Family Welfare, 1983), 2.
115 Ibid.
116 Ibid., 3–4.
117 MoHFW, 1983: *National Health Policy*, op. cit. Also see Duggal, "Historical Review of Health Policy Making", 33.
118 Duggal, "Historical Review of Health Policy Making", 33.
119 Mukhopadhyay, *Report of the Independent Commission*, 38.
120 Duggal, "Historical Review of Health Policy Making", 34.
121 MoHFW, NHP, 1983.
122 For details regarding the gross failure of the NHP 1983, see Mukhopadhyay, *Report of the Independent Commission*.
123 Duggal, "Historical Review of Health Policy Making", 33.
124 MoHFW, NHP, 1983.
125 Paria, *An Appeal*, 9. Also see Baru, *Private Health Care*, 52.
126 Meera Chatterjee, *Implementing Health Policy* (New Delhi: Manohar, 1988), 7.
127 Ibid., 1.
128 Ibid., 12–13.
129 Ibid., 125.
130 Ibid., 126.
131 Ibid., 126–27.
132 Interview with Dr Gauripada Dutta at East Nursing Home Private Limited, on 24.07.2007.
133 Chatterjee, *Implementing Health Policy*, 129–31.
134 Rao, *Do We Care?*, 14.
135 Duggal and Antia, "Health Financing in India", 56.
136 Planning Commission, *Government of India Seventh Five Year Plan 1985–90 Vol. II: Sectoral Programmes of Development* (New Delhi: Planning Commission, Government of India, 1990).
137 Shailendra Kumar Hooda, "Health System in Transition in India: Journey from State Provisioning to Privatization", *World Review of Political Economy* 11, no.

4 (Winter 2020): 508. (Hereafter cited as Hooda, "Health System in Transition in India").
138 Rao, *Do We Care?*, 17.

References

Alavi, Seema. "Unani Medicine in the Nineteenth-Century Public Sphere: Urdu Texts and Oudh Akbar". *Indian Economic and Social History Review* 42 (March 2005): 101–129.

Antia, Noshir, Seema Deodhar, and Nerges Mistry, eds. *Developing an Alternative Strategy for Achieving Health for All.* The ICSSR/ICMR model - The FRCH Experience. Pune: The Foundation for Research in Community Health, 2004.

Arnold, David. *Colonizing the Body: State Medicine and Epidemic Diseases in Nineteenth Century India*. Delhi: OUP, 1993.

Bagchi, Amiya, and Soman, Krishna, eds. *Maladies, Preventives and Curatives. Debates in Public Health Care.* Institute of Development Studies. Kolkata: Tulika Books, 2005.

Bala, Poonam. *Imperialism and Medicine in Bengal: A Socio-Historical Perspective*. New Delhi and London: Sage Publications, 1991.

Banerji, Debabar. "Political Dimensions of Health and Health Services". *Economic and Political Weekly* XIII, no. 22 (3 June 1978): 924–928.

Baru, Rama V., Arnab Acharya, Sanghmitra Acharya, A.K. Shiva Kumar, and K. Nagaraj. "Inequities to Access Health Services in India: Caste, Class, Region". *Economic and Political Weekly* 45, no. 38 (2010): 49–58.

Baru, Rama V., ed. *Medical Insurance Schemes for the Poor — Who Benefits*. New Delhi: Academic Foundation, 2015.

Baru, Rama V. *Private Health Care in India. Social Characteristics and Trends*. New Delhi: Sage Publications, 1998.

Basu, D.D. *Shorter Constitution of India*. Calcutta: S.C. Sarkar, 1981.

Bayley, C.A. *Empire and Information: Intelligence Gathering and Social Communication in India, 1780–1870*. Cambridge: Cambridge University Press, 1996.

Bennet, Sara, Barbara McPake, and Anne Mills, eds. *Private Health Providers: In Developing Countries-Serving the Public Interest?* London: Zed Books, 1997.

Berger, Rachel. *Ayurveda Made Modern: Political Histories of Indigenous Medicine in North India, 1900–1955.* Cambridge Imperial and Post-colonial Studies Series. New York: Palgrave Macmillan, 2013.

Berman, Peter, and M.E. Khan. *Paying for India's Health Care*. New Delhi: Sage Publications, 1993.

Biswanath, Paria. *An Appeal*. Kolkata: Medical Service Centre, 1985.

Borker, G. *Health in Independent India*. New Delhi: Ministry of Health, 1960.

Chakravarthy, Indira. "Role of World Health Organisation". *Economic and Political Weekly* 43, no. 47 (November:2008).

Chatterjee, Meera. *Implementing Health Policy*. Centre for Policy Research. New Delhi: Manohar, 1988.

Crawford, D.G. "Notes on the Early Hospitals of Calcutta". *Indian Medical Gazette* 38, no. 1 (1903): 3–7.

Dasgupta, Uma, ed. *Science and Modern India: An Institutional History, c 1784-c 1947*. Delhi: Centre for Studies in Civilizations, 2011.

Representatives from 134 countries 67 international organisations and many non governmental organisations. *Declaration of Alma-Ata International Conference on Primary Health Care, Alma-Ata*. USSR, 6–12 September 1978.

Duggal, Ravi. "Medical Education in India: Who Pays". *Radical Journal of Health* 3, no. 4 (March 1989): 5–12.

Duggal, Ravi, "Where Are We Today". Seminar Web Edition, Monthly Symposium, New Delhi, 2000.

Foucault, Michael. *The Birth of the Clinic: An Archaeology of Medical Perception*. New York: Vintage Books, 1975.

Foucault, Michael. "The Crisis of Medicine or the Crisis of Antimedicine?" English Translation: *Foucault Studies* 1 (2004): 5–19. Translated by Edgar C. Knowlton, Jr., William J. Kingand Clare O'Farrell.

Gangolli, Leena V., Duggal Ravi, and Shukla Abhay, eds. *Review of Healthcare in India*. Mumbai: Centre for Enquiry into Health and Allied Themes, 2005.

Government of India. *Health Survey and Development Committee (Bhore Committee) Report, Vol. 1–4*. New Delhi: Manager of Publications, 1946.

Government of India. *The Second Five Year Plan*. New Delhi: Planning Commission, 1956.

Government of India. *Third Five-Year Plan: A Draft Outline*. New Delhi: Planning Commission, 1960.

Government of India. *Report of the Health Survey and Planning Committee. (Mudaliar Committee)*. New Delhi: Ministry of Health, 1961.

Guha, Ratnabir. "Native Bodies, Medical Market and 'Conflicting' Medical 'Systems': Venereal Diseases and the 'Vernacularisation' of Western Medical Knowledge in Colonial Bengal". *Presidency Historical Review* 1, no. 1 (March 13, 2015): 11–18.

Hodges, Sarah and Mohan Rao. *Public Health and Private Wealth: Stem Cells, Surrogates and Other Strategic Bodies*. Delhi: Oxford University Press, 2016.

Hooda, Shailender Kumar. "Health System in Transition in India: Journey from State Provisioning to Privatization". *World Review of Political Economy* 11, no. 4, (2020).

http://nhp.gov.in/health-policies.

ICSSR/ICMR. *Health for All: An Alternative Strategy*. Pune: Indian Institute of Education, 1981.

Illich, Ivan. *Medical Nemesis: The Expropriation of Health*. London: Calder and Boyars, 1974.

Interview with Dr Gauripada Dutta at East Nursing Home Private Limited, Kolkata, 24 July 2007.

Jeffrey, Roger. *Politics of Health in India*. Berkeley, CA: University of California Press, 1988.

Kapilashrami, Anuj, and Rama V. Baru, eds. *Global Health Governance and Commercialisation of Public Health in India: Actors, Institutions and Dialectics of Global and Local*. Edinburgh: Routledge, 2019.

Kosambi, D.D. *An Introduction to the Study of Indian History*. Bombay: Popular Prakashan, 1975, revised 2nd edition.

MoHFW. *National Health Policy*. New Delhi: Govt. of India, Ministry of Health & Family Welfare, 1983.

Muir, D.M. "Notes on the Origin of the Presidency General Hospital Calcutta". *Indian Medical Gazzette* 38, no. 1 (1903): 43–44, 73.

Mukharji, Projit Bihari. *Nationalizing the Body: The Medical Market, Print and Daktari Medicine*. New York: Anthem Press, 2009.

Mukhopadhyay, Alok. *Report of the Independent Commission on Health in India*. New Delhi: Voluntary Health Associations of India, 1997.

Palit, Chittyabrata, and Achintya Dutta. *History of Medicine in India: The Medical Encounter*. Delhi: Kalpaaz Publication, 2005.

Pati, Biswamaoy, and Harrison Mark. *Health Medicine and Empire Perspectives on Colonial Medicine*. New Delhi: Oxford University Press, 2001.

Planning Commission. *Government of India, Fourth Five Year Plan*. New Delhi: Planning Commission, Government of India, 1969.

Planning Commission. *Government of India, Sixth Five Year Plan 1980–85*. New Delhi: Planning Commission, Government of India, 1985.

Planning Commission. *Government of India Seventh Five Year Plan 1985–90 Vol. II: Sectoral Programmes of Development*. New Delhi: Planning Commission, Government of India, 1990.

Porter, Roy. *Health for Sale: Quackery in England, 1660–85*. Manchester: Manchester University Press, 1989.

Prasad, Purendra, and Jessani Amar, eds. *Equity and Access: Health Care Studies in India*. New Delhi: OUP, 2018.

Qadeer, Imrana, Kasturi Sen, and K.R. Nayar, eds. *Public Health and Poverty of Reforms*. New Delhi: Sage Publications, 2001.

Rao, K.N. "Public Health and Health Services". *Encyclopaedia of Social Work, Vol. I*. New Delhi: Publication Division, 1995.

Rao, K. Sujatha. Do We Care? India's Health System. New Delhi: OUP, 2020.

Sathia, Suthanthiraveeran. *The Five Years Plans in India, Overview of Public Health Policies*. https://www.researchgate.net/publication/327238255, 2011.

Sharma, Madhuri. *Indigenous and Western Medicine in Colonial India, Culture and Environment in South Asia*. New Delhi: Foundation Books, 2012.

Sigerist, Henry E. *A History of Medicine: Early Greek, Hindu, and Persian Medicine, Vol. 2*. New York: OUP, 1961.

Subramanian, S.V., and V.R. Madhavan, eds. *Heritage of the Tamils: Siddha Medicine Madras*. Chennai, Tamilnadu: International Institute of Tamil Studies, 1983.

Sujatha, V. *Sociology of Health and Medicine: New Perspectives*. New Delhi: OUP, 2014.

Tata, J.R.D., G.D. Birla, P. Thakurdas, K. Lalbhai, A. Dalal, L. Shri Ram, J. Mathai, and A.D. Shroff. *Brief Memorandum Outlining a Plan of Economic Development for India (Bombay Plan)*. London: Penguin Books, 1946.

Thapar, Romila. *Ashoka and the Decline of the Mauryas*. Oxford: OUP, 1973.

Twaddle, Andrew C. *Health Care Reform around the World*. Connecticut: Auburn House, 2002.

World Health Organisation. *Thirty-Fourth World Health Assembly*, Geneva, 4–22 May, 1981. Verbatim Records of Plenary Meetings and Reports of Committees. Geneva: WHO, 1981.

2 Changing Paradigm in Health Sector (Plans, Policies and Reports)

Mid-1980s to 2000s

The Eighth Five Year Plan, in keeping with the selective healthcare approach, adopted a new slogan – instead of Health for All by 2000 AD it chose to emphasize Health for the Underprivileged. Simultaneously it continued the support for privatization, 'In accordance with the new policy of the government to encourage private initiatives, private hospitals and clinics will be supported subject to maintenance of minimum standards and suitable returns for the tax incentives'.[1]

Parallely, the advent of the wave of liberalism in India in the post-1991 era had three characteristics that questioned the state's ability to provide an alternative mode of service delivery: marginalization of state, primacy to markets and ceding space to NGOs. As a result, the gap between rich and poor did not exhibit a positive picture and poverty did not decline. Nehru's brand of socialism had indeed become passé.[2]

Until the early 1980s the state encouraged private nursing homes and small and medium hospitals to supplement government healthcare. Private healthcare was scattered and fragmented and did account for a large-scale healthcare provider.[3]

In 1991, there was a drastic cut in the central government budgetary allocation for healthcare, which favoured the establishment of private hospitals in India. Successive governments encouraged the growth of the private sector in various ways, such as releasing the prime building land at low rates, providing an exemption from taxes and duties for importing drugs, high-tech medical equipment and so forth.[4]

Thus, there was a gradual paradigmatic shift in the domain of healthcare services where healthcare itself was commodified. Hospitals became lucrative commercial enterprises, medical education became investment destinations and patients became clients. Moreover, the shift from the family doctor to a professionally managed health machine was also inevitable. In the face of technological innovation in medical devices, the discovery of new drugs, rapid changes in disease profile towards non-communicable diseases that required better diagnostic tools, more sophisticated laboratory facilities and institutionalized treatment, healthcare became specialist dependent, organizationally structured and resource intensive. By 1990, private players accounted for 58 per cent of hospitals and 29 per cent of beds.[5]

DOI: 10.4324/9781003169475-3

Meagre government spending on healthcare led to the abandoning of the vision of Comprehensive Primary Healthcare (Health for All by 2000 AD). With the transformation in the health policies and programmes and in the patterns of allocation, the exogeneous factors started playing a dominant role. With international and bilateral funding of some of the programmes, there is a gross distortion of priorities in health development and disease control.[6]

Certain distinct patterns can be identified regarding the volume of funds, main funding agencies (both bilateral and multilateral), the period of funding and the type of programmes being funded. During the 1970s and 1980s, foreign funding was being channelized through bilateral agencies. Minor contributions also came from Christian organizations based mainly in Europe. There was a major shift in funding patterns from the mid-eighties onwards. Bilateral commitments decreased, and multilateral agencies (like World Bank and IMF) became major investors in the health programmes of the country. Moreover, it has been noticed that the increasing role of international financial organizations in health and development policies has resulted in growing inequalities in health.[7]

With the coming of the World Bank on the stage in 1993, three key features had been clearly discerned:[8]

- The concept of an essential health service package as opposed to the grand vision of comprehensive primary care articulated at Alma-Ata.
- Confining the role of government in implementing selective disease control programmes justified on principles of disability adjusted life years (DALYs).
- Allowing markets to provide hospital and medical care with government engagement on the basis of public–private partnerships.

This vertical intervention programme of the World Bank has to be seen within the Structural Adjustment Programme (SAP), where the investment in social sectors is viewed as important for cushioning the vulnerable sections from the impact of the SAP. The World Bank emphasized building health infrastructure and preventing and controlling communicable diseases. Thus, the World Bank has emerged as the single largest fund loaning agency during the early nineties. The World Bank package on communicable diseases focuses primarily on AIDS, malaria, tuberculosis (TB) and blindness. This was made amply clear by the fact that between 1990 and 1993, World Bank funding for AIDS went up from Rs 400 lakh to Rs 5800 lakhs while the budget for malaria declined by 38 per cent during the same period. Before the 1990s, the World Bank was primarily involved in population projects and nutrition programmes.[9]

External assistance in India has been through centrally sponsored programmes for communicable diseases and family welfare. In the seventies and eighties, bilateral agencies focused on leprosy and malaria among communicable diseases. The funding for malaria was mainly from the USA in the seventies while European bilateral agencies mainly funded leprosy, tuberculosis and family welfare programmes. Most of the external funding was spent on these areas. The

Indian Government has recently restricted external assistance for centrally sponsored programmes.[10]

There has been a perceptible shift in the pattern of external health funding between 1985 and 1995. In the 1970s bilateral agencies largely emphasized the supply of contraceptives, technology for sterilization, training, consultancy and research. Most of the area projects failed to achieve results. The outcome of evaluations has been ignored. During the late 1980s and 1990s, there was a systematic shift to cover all the area projects under a model plan, and hence the focus on infrastructure building.[11]

In 1981, the World Bank provided US$ 33 million, which rose to US$ 263 million in 1990. Before the SAP period, World Bank funding was generally given as grants. However, during the SAP period, soft loans were given for various health programmes. Grants could directly subsidize the service, whereas in soft loans, such a means of deficit financing implied later repayments.[12] Accordingly, under the Health Sector Reform (HSR), several states availed of loans. Although such strengthening of infrastructure capacity was undertaken during the decade after 1995 in states like Andhra Pradesh, Karnataka, West Bengal, Uttar Pradesh and Rajasthan, institutional deliveries and hospital care for the poor did not bring about many desired changes. In such a scenario, India plays a very small role in setting its own priorities and has to accept conditionalities. While AIDS gets priority funding from the World Bank, it is still not a major cause of mortality in India; other major diseases (like tuberculosis, diarrhoea and malaria) which cause high morbidity and mortality get less importance.[13]

Thus, from 1990 to 2000, the influence of the World Bank, WHO and donor agencies on policy formulation was strong, though the share of their funding was less than 2 per cent of the total health spending. Complex health problems were simplified into single-lined technical solutions – DOTS for TB, immunization for infant mortality, early diagnosis and distribution of chloroquine tablets for malaria and cataract surgeries for blindness. Health problems of India are being addressed through technological solutions while ignoring the social dimension of disease causation and neglecting the importance of social determinants.[14]

In family welfare, the emphasis is on infrastructure building, mainly sub-centres (SCs). But the issue is when the external funding stops how the states will run these sub-centres.[15]

Another crucial development of neoliberal health policies in India was the introduction of user fees. In 1987, the World Bank, in its report 'Financing Health Services in Developing Countries: An Agenda for Reform', recommended the introduction of user fees in government healthcare services, steering the debate towards the financial efficiency of these institutions rather than addressing the financial crisis of the poor households and critically analyzing the financial schemes of the government healthcare system. Several policy documents of the World Bank also recommended the introduction of user charges in the public hospitals of India.

In the context of making the public sector hospitals autonomous, proponents of user fees see it as a revenue mobilizing avenue. However, revenue generated from a user fee has not been very encouraging. In a district hospital in West Bengal, from 2002/2003 to 2005/2006, the share of user charges to the total expenditure showed a decline from 2.1 per cent to 1.8 per cent and the major share of revenue was generated from diagnostic services.[16]

The World Bank pushed the private sector agenda, introducing the concept of public–private partnership (PPP). Justified on the grounds of organizational efficiencies, the concepts of 'outsourcing' and contracting services such as sanitation, laundry, diet and the delivery of allied services took root, gradually expanding to co-opt NGOs and private sector care providers as partners. There was a clear shift towards the growth of curative (tertiary) services with a strong commercial focus on the neglect of primary health services. Attempts were initiated to take over hospital lands for other purposes, non-renewal of land leases to charity hospitals, attempts to hand over primary health centres to private organizations and so on were some major reforms that occurred in the last two decades. These measures have been justified by the state as being reform measures to increase the viability of healthcare services.[17]

From the First Plan onwards, the government had elicited support and cooperation of 'for-profit' and 'non-profit' sectors in the malaria and family planning programmes. Initially the government sought the support of NGOs at the primary level for community mobilization and education. But later these collaborations extended to the for-profit sector and several other national health programmes. Private and non-governmental collaborations have largely been for creating awareness and demand for family planning services through community mobilization. Only a small proportion of private practitioners and clinics were involved in providing contraception and abortion services. The state provided subsidies in the form of devices and monetary incentives to these sectors for providing services. It is during the last two decades that the concept of PPPs has been introduced into health programmes. The distinction between the PPPs of the 1990s and the earlier forms of collaboration is that the former conceptualizes both partners as equal and is arbitrated through a formal memorandum of understanding (MoU), while in the latter the role of non-state players was peripheral to the programme. During the mid-1980s the idea of PPPs got introduced into several disease control and Reproductive and Child Health (RCH) programmes.[18]

During the Eighth Plan, resources were provided to set up the Education Commission for Health Sciences, and a few states have even set up the University for Health Sciences as per the recommendations of the Bajaj Committee report of 1987. This initiative was to bring all health sciences together, provide for continuing medical education and improve medical and health education through such integration.[19]

An Expert Committee on Public Health Systems was formed to make a thorough appraisal of public health programmes, and it found that we were facing a resurgence of most communicable diseases and there was a need to drastically improve disease surveillance in the country.

The Ninth Five Year Plan proposed to set up at the district level a strong detection cum response system for rapid containment of any outbreaks that may occur.

The recommendations of the committee mentioned above formed the basis of the Ninth Plan health sector strategy to revitalize the public health system in the country to respond to its healthcare needs in these changed times. The Plan also proposed horizontal integration of all vertical programmes at the district level to increase their effectiveness and facilitate allocative efficiencies. The Ninth Plan also reviewed the 1983 National Health Policy in the context of its objectives and goals and concluded that a reappraisal and reformulation of the National Health Policy (NHP) was necessary so that a reliable and relevant policy framework was available for not only improving healthcare but also measuring and monitoring the healthcare delivery systems and health status of the population in the next two decades. This Plan also reviewed the population policy and the family planning programme. In this review too it went back to the Bhore Committee report and said that the core of this programme was maternal and child health services. Assuring antenatal care, safe delivery and immunization is critical to reducing infant and maternal mortality and this in turn has a bearing on contraception use and fertility rates. In the midst of all this, the National Population Policy was announced with a lot of fanfare in the middle of 2000. It is definitely an improvement from its predecessors, but the underlying element remains population control and not population welfare.[20]

Thus the Eight (1992–1997) and Ninth (1997–2002) Plans highlighted the following points:[21]

- Increased involvement of voluntary and private organizations, self-help groups and social marketing organization in improving access to healthcare.
- Contracting in and out of clinical and non-clinical services. NGO sectors to support the government in handling RCH services like providing transport for emergency obstetric care for which funds would be devolved at the village level and PPPs introduced in several states.
- Preparation of Information, Education and Communication (IEC) material and social marketing of contraceptives has been handed over to the NGO sector.

In 1993, the World Bank published a report on 'Investing in Health',[22] which acknowledged the role of government efforts in improving health outcomes and argued that the public healthcare system in developing nations was confronted with several challenges in the areas of efficiency and equity. It insisted that government involvement in the healthcare and health insurance sectors had only a limited role to play and that the government should restrict its role in these areas. The report rejected the idea of healthcare as a public good and proposed that healthcare provisions were a matter of individuals and families, with their strikingly different health needs, and they should be able to choose freely.[23]

The second report in 2001 titled 'India: Raising the Sights: Better Health Systems for India's Poor'[24] highlighted that India's healthcare system was at a crossroads. Its ability to combat infant mortality, communicable diseases and malnutrition was being stretched. At the same time, the system faced emerging demands for better services and for more attention to be paid to chronic diseases of adulthood. India's underfunded public sector and extensive but largely unaccountable private sector could not hope to meet the country's enormous, growing and shifting healthcare needs. The country needed to promote its private health sector and in this way, to take better advantage of the supposed capacity of the private sector to deliver better services and outcomes for all regions and socio-economic groups.

Thus, the period from the mid-1980s to early 2000s shows that the government healthcare system grew weak by the 1990s and deteriorated further since 2000, with the retreat of the welfare state. Despite growing health needs, the state did not increase its budgetary allocation; rather it introduced partial user charges, created paying and non-paying wards in public hospitals and so on. Also, referral services, from primary to secondary and tertiary levels became weak links and hospitals increasingly levied charges for items such as drugs and surgical supplies. As a result, the cost of healthcare, particularly for the labouring poor, increased continuously. These processes also accelerated the flight to private healthcare services and decline in the utilization of public services.[25]

Healthcare Policies and Developments from 2000s Onwards

On the eve of the Tenth Plan, the Draft National Health Policy 2001 was announced, and for the first time, feedback was invited from the public. 'Universal, comprehensive, primary healthcare services', the NHP 1983 goal, was not even mentioned in the NHP 2001 but the latter bravely acknowledged that the public healthcare system was grossly short of defined requirements, functioning was far from satisfactory, morbidity and mortality due to easily curable diseases continued to be unacceptably high and resource allocations were generally insufficient.[26]

The policy is focused on those diseases which are principally contributing to the disease burden – TB, malaria and blindness from the category of historical diseases and HIV/AIDS from the category of 'newly emerging diseases'. This is not to say that other items contributing to the disease burden of the country will be ignored but only that the resources, as also the principal focus of the public health administration, will recognize certain relative priorities. It is unnecessary to labour the point that under the umbrella of the macro-policy prescriptions in this document, governments and private sector programme planners will have to design separate schemes, tailor-made to the health needs of women, children, geriatrics, tribals and other socio-economically underserved sections. An adequately robust disaster management plan has to be in place to effectively cope with situations arising from natural and man-made calamities.[27]

One nagging imperative, which has influenced every aspect of this policy, is the need to ensure that 'equity' in the health sector stands as an independent goal. In any future evaluation of its success or failure, NHP 2002 would wish to be measured against this equity norm rather than any other aggregated financial norm for the health sector. Consistent with the primacy given to 'equity', a marked emphasis has been provided in the policy for expanding and improving the primary health facilities, including the new concept of the provisioning of essential drugs through central funding.[28]

In principle, this policy welcomes the participation of the private sector in all areas of health activities – primary, secondary or tertiary. However, looking at past experiences of the private sector, it can reasonably be expected that its contribution would be substantial in the urban primary sector and the tertiary sector and moderate in the secondary sector. This policy envisaged the enactment of suitable legislation for regulating minimum infrastructure and quality standards in clinical establishments/medical institutions by 2003. Also, statutory guidelines for the conduct of clinical practice and delivery of medical services were targeted to be developed over the same period. With the acquiring of experience in the setting and enforcing of minimum quality standards, the policy envisaged graduation to a scheme of quality accreditation of clinical establishments/medical institutions for the information of the citizenry.[29]

The key features of the National Health Policy 2002:[30]

- Primary healthcare approach.
- Decentralized public health system.
- Convergence of all health programmes under a single field umbrella.
- Strengthening and extending public health services.
- Enhanced contribution of private and NGO sectors in healthcare delivery.
- Increase in public spending for healthcare.

The NHP 2002 reiterated its commitment to achieving a more equitable access to health services across the social and geographical expanse of the country through comprehensive PHC services. However, in practice, the state gradually divested its responsibility even from the curative care as a part of the economic reforms. This led to the unfettered growth of the private hospitals that found it lucrative to adopt the tertiary care model. The private sector grew without adequate regulation and eventually resulted in the corporatization of healthcare. With good quality health services becoming unaffordable and inaccessible, curative healthcare today is left to the initiative of the patient reinforcing the neoliberal idea of individualizing healthcare.[31]

The policy document talks of integration of vertical programmes, strengthening of the infrastructure, providing universal health services, decentralization of the healthcare delivery system through Panchayati Raj Institutions (PRIs) and other autonomous institutions and regulation of private healthcare but fails to indicate how it achieves the goals.[32]

Soon after the second NHP announcement, the Government of India in 2003 implemented the Fiscal Responsibility and Budget Management (FRBM) Act. The purpose of the FRBM Act was to force the central and state governments to reduce fiscal and revenue deficits, either by increasing their revenue resources or by restructuring/curtailing overall public expenditure. Since the federal nature of the country means that most of the revenue-generating capacities lie with the central government, the state governments followed the route of expenditure curtailment, with the health sector bearing the brunt of the cutbacks. At this particular time, the all-state average health spending fell significantly, to around 3.4 per cent of total budget outlays.[33]

Thus, the second National Health Policy was called realistic and equitable. The BJP-led National Democratic Alliance (NDA), which came to power in 1999, condemned the policies of the previous government. Although there were some people-oriented promises, these were not implemented.

World Bank–IMF-generated policies on healthcare failed to bring about any positive outcome by 2004. The post-liberalization rhetoric, namely, 'New Public Health' (NPH) has replaced the primary healthcare approach. The NPH is in harmony with the World Bank's essential package of services. It has eliminated the concept of planning for population as a national agenda and talks of healthy 'cities' and 'communities', thereby shifting responsibility to the local organizations. The NPH approach reduces the role of the state and makes it seek partners in the private, corporate and NGO sectors. The primary healthcare approach emphasizes on equitably distributed health resources and social measures, whereas NPH is only interested in 'health status'.[34]

In eight states, substantial investments were mobilized from the World Bank to upgrade, strengthen and establish hospitals at the district, sub-district and block levels. Under these projects, the comprehensive definition of the primary health infrastructure got a further distortion with the community health centres (CHCs) rechristened as first referral centres (FRUs), divorcing them from their contextual framework. In Andhra Pradesh, Karnataka, Punjab, etc., the World Bank-funded CHCs were brought under the administrative control of autonomous directorates dealing with secondary level hospitals, while those CHCs not covered under the project were continued to be administered by the Director of Health Services. An evaluation report of West Bengal, Andhra Pradesh, Karnataka and Punjab showed that while these projects were successful in improving the quality of care in urban and semi-urban areas, an expected outcome, such as, for example, an increase in institutional deliveries was not realized. Had the focus been on establishing the referral system and linkages with the other World Bank-assisted disease control and RCH projects, investments made for strengthening the health systems would have had a measurable impact on reducing maternal, neonatal and infant deaths or deaths due to malaria and TB, which require hospitalization. This experience clearly demonstrates that a mere increase in investments in infrastructure does not automatically translate into better public health outcomes. It also underscores the urgent need for conceptual clarity on the expectations of the organizational structures that have been established and the urgent need for standardization of facilities across the country. Shortage of funds has been primarily responsible for the non-availability of facilities in accordance with the norms set by the government and inadequate provisioning of critical inputs such as drugs, equipment, facilities such as operation theatre, etc. Free services to a select list of interventions were an inadequate response to the unfolding social crisis with people either denying themselves timely care or getting into indebtedness due to their ability to pay.

Several studies estimated that 20 per cent of people did not seek treatment even when they needed to on account of financial reasons. Moreover, 32.45 million people were being pushed below the poverty line every year because of medical expenses.[35]

Due to lack of budgets and the pressure to achieve targets, several states upgraded the two-roomed sub-centres to PHCs. With no place for laboratory, examination, pharmacy, etc., most are non-functional. There are PHCs with over 33 sub-centres and there are sub-centres which cover over 200 habitations. It is estimated that 25 per cent of the people in Madhya Pradesh and Orissa and 11 per cent in Uttar Pradesh could not access medical care due to locational reasons. What emerges from the health outcomes are poor. This shows that it is not the mere establishment of a physical facility but a combination of factors such as distance, availability and quality of skills, adequacy of infrastructure and access to alternative sources of care that seem to influence health-seeking behaviour and determine outcomes which have been captured by a set of indicators such as complete immunization, percentage of those severely malnourished, full antenatal coverage, safe and institutional deliveries and finally, the infant mortality rate (IMR) and the under-five mortality rate. While it is clear that infrastructure development had little linkage to goal setting, it is also seen that policy interventions per se often lacked focus, were not based on hard evidence and had weak institutional capacity to translate policy into action. It was thus clear that the strategy of starving the public health sector of funds resulted in the collapse of the slender social security net the poor had, particularly in rural areas, forcing them to go to private clinics for every blood test or treatment of fevers.[36]

With the coming of the Tenth Plan, focus was made on improving the efficiency of the existing healthcare system, quality of care, logistics of supplies of drugs and diagnostics and promotion of the rational use of drugs. The focus was also on evolving, implementing and evaluating systems of healthcare financing so that essential healthcare based on need is available to all at an affordable cost. The reductions in fertility, mortality and population growth rates were also the major objectives during this period. The Tenth Plan also proposed the redesigning of the Universal Health Insurance scheme introduced in 2003 to make it exclusive for below poverty level people with a reduced premium and introduction of Group Health Insurance scheme for members of self-help groups.[37]

The key features of the Tenth Plan (2002–2007)[38] are as follows:

- Increased involvement of voluntary and private organizations, self-help groups and social marketing organization in improving access to healthcare.
- Contracting in and out of clinical and non-clinical services.
- NGO sectors to support the government in handling RCH services like providing transport for emergency obstetric care for which funds would be devolved at the village level and PPPs introduced in several states.
- Preparation of IEC material and social marketing of contraceptives has been handed over to the NGO sector.

In the second phase of Health Sector Reforms, the World Health Organization proposed that the higher growth rates in economies in distress through commoditization of health services and its techno-centric growth are more desirable than improving equity in public health. The slogan of inclusive development was used by the government's flagship programme, the National Rural Health Mission (NRHM), in 2005 promising full coverage to the rural population. The NRHM has been a noble experiment in the direction of improving status of health in the country. As per the Constitution of India, health has been a state subject but the Centre always recognized the need to support state health action to provide equitable and effective services to people belonging to different regions and social groups. The NRHM (2005–2007) was launched on 12 April 2005 by the Prime Minister to improve the status of health services in India. It is based on the understanding that under the prevailing circumstances, States required additional funds and technical and institutional support from the Centre to improve the health status of their population. The stated aim of the NRHM was to provide accessible, affordable and accountable quality services to the rural population with concentration on 18 'Special Focus States' and the poor. These states included the Empowered Action Group States, States of the North-East, Jammu and Kashmir and Himachal Pradesh.[39]

It is notable that apart from providing financial support, several new institutional changes were envisaged. These included communitization of funds, flexible financing, improved management through capacity building, improved monitoring against standards and innovations in human resource management. Provisions of untied funds, involvement of PRIs, PPPs and convergence of the health sector and a wide range of other determinants of health (e.g., water, sanitation, education, nutrition, social and gender equality) were created to develop 'a fully functional health system at all levels, from the village to the district'.[40]

Quoting the Independence Day speech, 2012, of the Prime Minister, the Twelfth Five Year Plan document notes that the success of the NRHM shows the way for converting the NRHM into the National Health Mission (NHM), which would cover both rural and urban areas. Thus, an impression was created that the NRHM has been quite successful in achieving its goals. It was extended up to 2017.[41]

This NRHM aimed at improving rural health by targeting phased increase in the funding for health up to 2–3 per cent of the gross domestic product (GDP) in coming years. A critical review of the NRHM also tries to correct most of the shortcomings of previous programmes, i.e., inappropriate training, lack of technical guidance, supervision and coordination and poor community participation.[42] Thus, the objectives of the NRHM were decentralization and community engagement through community health workers (CHWs) and other community-based initiatives and to revitalize the rural primary healthcare system.

In the NRHM, the commitment of the government was palpable and categorical as the programme was time-bound, with clear objectives and achievable goals. All these factors made the NRHM a different programme from the previous ones. The desire for achievable targets was reflected in the acceptance of Indian Public

Health Standards (IPHS) for CHCs accepting that BIS standards were very much resource-oriented and difficult to achieve under the present conditions of the health system in India.[43]

It seems that before planning the NRHM, the target of meeting the Millennium Development Goals (MDGs), of which India is a signatory, was also kept in the mind, as the goals under the NRHM were similar to what has been envisaged in MDGs. Another pertinent point to be noted is that the NRHM addressed two of the four major problems identified in the UN Millennium Project and associated with the poor development of the countries. First is the problem of poor governance and second policy neglect in the form of unawareness of what to do or neglect of core public issues. Both of these may be taken as right steps in the direction of achieving the MDGs.[44]

The NRHM had a central functionary named Accredited Social Health Activist (ASHA). ASHA is a resurrection of the earlier CHW or Village Health Guide (VHG), both almost 30-year-old schemes. Agreeably, ASHA is a newer and modified version of CHW, but lessons learnt from older schemes or causes attributed to her failure, i.e., improper selection, inadequate training and demand of fee for service have been incorporated in the scheme. At the same time ASHA is an activist and not a worker in the health system as the previous CHW or VHGs. Besides, ASHA is more similar to the very successful and concept of 'barefoot doctors' in China. ASHA appears to be an appropriate mix of the CHWs and the idea of barefoot doctors.[45]

ASHA is the main stakeholder in the programme, but it has not been planned what should be done if an ASHA leaves the health system. The selection of ASHA is rigorous and time consuming. Besides, she has to be given sufficient training to function properly so it would take approximately one year for selecting another similar functionary. Strategies to sustain ASHA, along with a contingency plan for a situation when an ASHA leaves the system prematurely, need to be developed. Secondly, dependency of ASHA on Anganwadi workers (AWWs) and auxilliary nurse midwives (ANMs) is likely and it seems that there is hardly any freedom for her to work independently. It may be detrimental to the system in a way that other functionaries might start delegating their work to ASHA. The work responsibility of ASHA and other workers need to be more clearly defined and mutually exclusive.

The NRHM discusses the making of the health system functional from the sub-centre level. An untied fund of Rs 10,000 has been widely publicized as a component of strengthening the sub-centres. While it is a well-known fact that most sub-centres are in operation without any available buildings, priority should be given on finding a building for sub-centres and allocation of Rs 10,000 would be useful only when there is infrastructure available to carry out activities. The strengthening of sub-centres is of paramount importance and allocation of this money is good but it does not solve the most important issue of the building for the sub-centres, as these are the point of first contact between the community and the health system and should be presentable enough.[46]

The Rogi Kalyan Samiti (RKS) scheme was started in Madhya Pradesh, a low performance state, and was very successful. This simply conveys that we need not to be unnecessarily cynical but try to replicate it all over the country. It is a good step, which can be extended to all hospitals in our country in future.[47]

However, the UN MDGs addressed only 'extreme poverty' that was to be halved by the target year 2015; universal 'primary' education and not 'secondary' education was the target; child mortality was to be reduced to two-third and the maternal mortality ratio (MMR) to three-fourth; human immunodeficiency virus infection/acquired immunodeficiency syndrome, tuberculosis and malaria were to be combated in collaboration with the pharmaceutical companies and sanitation and drinking water supply were to be improved with better technology. The NRHM that was to work towards the MDGs, succeeded only in narrowing the focus of primary health centres (PHCs) to reproductive healthcare, could not integrate vertical programmes and fragmented the different levels of care by diverting referrals primarily to the private sector. It thus remained far from being genuinely inclusive. However, it focused mainly on maternal and child health and did not cover many other health conditions such as hypertension, diabetes or mental illness, which are now widely prevalent and has not yet integrated many vertical infectious disease control programmes. It therefore remained an incomplete programme of primary healthcare.[48]

A review indicated some success in improving drug supplies, increasing the number of functional PHCs in addition to creating ASHAs. It pointed out that the NRHM never received the required financial support of Rs 900 per capita and functions with an allocation of only Rs 270 per capita. This is in contrast to India's defence expenditure being Rs 164,415.49 crores for the year 2011–2012 inevitably impacting inputs into welfare and bringing health expenditure to Rs 28,353.06 crore for the same period.[49]

The NRHM failed to achieve its stated objectives. The most important lesson that ought to be learnt is that 'the health of the people is not a standalone phenomenon that can be improved through healthcare alone. It requires a comprehensive action plan encompassing food security, employment and poverty alleviation as well'.[50]

Another significant development in healthcare was the introduction of Rashtriya Swasthya Bima Yojana (RSBY). In recent years, several developing countries have introduced tax-financed health insurance coverage to their poor populations. India too, joined this effort in 2008, with the Indian Ministry of Labour and Employment (MoL&E) launching the RSBY to protect poor Indian households from financial risks associated with hospitalization expenses.[51]

Earlier, government has tried to provide health insurance to the resource-poor communities through different central or state schemes. However, these did not achieve the intended objectives due to a number of design- and implementation-related problems. India has Social Health Insurance (SHI) schemes like Employees' State Insurance (ESI) or the Central Government Health Scheme (CGHS), but these cover only those people who are employed in the formal sector apart from these, there were certain state-specific schemes.[52]

General Insurance Companies (GICs), established by the government in 1973, offer 'Mediclaim' policy through four major government-owned GICs. It covers hospitalization expenses, however with numerous exclusions criteria, which make it unviable from the patients' perspective. Moreover, it is not always cashless due to which poor people find it difficult to join. It offers reimbursement of expenses; delay in reimbursement is its major criticism.[53]

The RSBY is a centrally sponsored scheme that was implemented by the MoL&E from 2008 under the Unorganized Workers' Social Security Act 2008 to provide health insurance coverage to Below Poverty Line (BPL) families. Initially, the scheme was designed for BPL families but later it included 11 other categories of unorganized workers (UOWs) (MGNREGA workers, construction workers, domestic workers, sanitation workers, mine workers, licensed railway porters, street vendors, beedi workers, rickshaw pullers, ragpickers and auto/ taxi drivers). The scheme has now been transferred to the Ministry of Health and Family Welfare on an 'as is where is' basis with effect from 1 April 2015. Each family enrolled in the scheme is entitled to hospitalization benefits of up to Rs 30,000 per annum including maternity benefits on a family floater basis (a unit of five) in government empanelled hospitals (both private and public). Pre-existing conditions are covered from day one and there is no age limit. Transportation costs up to Rs 100 are also provisioned under the scheme. The scheme is implemented at the state level through a contractual arrangement between insurance companies and state government represented by the State Nodal Agency (SNA). At present the SNA is primarily responsible for overseeing the implementation of the RSBY at the state level, which includes managing the process of bidding, selection of insurance companies, overseeing the enrolment process, supporting the empanelment of providers, redressal of grievances and periodic review of the scheme on the ground. With effect from 2015 to 2016, the central government bears 60 per cent of insurance premium costs and the remaining cost is borne by the state government. In the case of North Eastern and three Himalayan states, the sharing pattern shifts to 90 per cent of support of the insurance premium cost from the Centre. In respect of union territories (without legislature), the central government share is 100 per cent, while in those with legislature, the central share will be 60 per cent. The Senior Citizen Health Insurance Scheme (SCHIS) provides insurance cover to senior citizens (aged 60 years and above) as a top-up over the existing RSBY scheme and has been implemented w.e.f. 1 April 2016. It will provide an enhanced coverage up to Rs 30,000 per senior citizen in the eligible family. The premium of the scheme would be met from the Senior Citizens Welfare Fund administered by the Ministry of Social Justice and Empowerment. The premium for the implementation of SCHIS will be paid by the Centre and States in the ratio 60:40 except the North Eastern states and three Himalayan states where it is 90:10.[54] By September 2016, more than 41 million families (about 150 million people) out of a targeted 65 million families were enrolled in RSBY.[55]

Several studies[56] have been undertaken on the impact of RSBY on the Indian population. However, it has been inferred that overall analysis shows that RSBY has not provided any significant financial protection for poor households. Drug expenditures do not provide the full story on why these impacts are small. The burden of outpatient expenditures that account for the bulk of out-of-pocket

(OOP) expenditure healthcare spending is mostly unaffected and utilization of outpatient care may even have increased on account of RSBY.[57]

The NSSO-CES analyses for the year 2007–2008 and 2009–2010 showed that RSBY was yet to provide benefits to the resource-poor households in terms of increased utilization of healthcare services, particularly for institutional care. It also shows that there are a number of issues related to design and implementation of the scheme, which may hinder it from achieving its intended objective of providing financial security from catastrophic health expenses to those families for whom the programme is meant for.[58]

The lack of health infrastructures in rural areas is a stumbling block for RSBY. As a result, in states like West Bengal, Bihar, Uttar Pradesh, Jharkhand and Chhattisgarh new private hospitals were set up with least-trained medical staff who performed complicated surgeries using non-sterilized surgical equipment and spurious drugs causing deaths of a huge number of patients. As a result, up to 2014, more than 250 hospitals were de-empanelled from the scheme due to fraud.[59]

Moreover, unnecessary investigations and invasive procedures unethically increased the profitability of the empanelled private hospitals but cause a greater damage to the healthy individuals. An estimate in 2012 found that nearly 7000 women had got their uterus removed under RSBY over a period of 30 months. RSBY only covers in-patient treatment. As two-thirds of the health expenditure was 'out of the pocket', RSBY failed to protect the labouring poor. Furthermore, under RSBY, patients were asked to buy medicines from private medical stores. Although the card holders were entitled to avail of hospital services throughout the country, their claim for treatments was not provided when they were away from their home state.[60]

Thus, RSBY in reality strengthened the platform for the private healthcare sector to flourish and challenged the treatment of patients who are the victims of increasing unethical practices in healthcare.

Meanwhile, the Eleventh Five Year Plan (2007–2012) was announced and it bemoaned the sorry state of affairs of the healthcare delivery system in India. The public healthcare system in many states was in shambles. Extreme inequalities and disparities persisted both in terms of access to healthcare as well as health outcome. The Plan deplored the critical shortage of health personnel, particularly doctors and nurses, poor working conditions and inadequate incentives and the low utilization of the meagre facilities in government hospitals. Government hospitals at all levels presented a picture of neglect and decline.[61]

The role of healthcare in economic development has received increasing attention in recent years. There is a general agreement that economic growth is not merely a function of incremental capital–output ratio. Investment in human development – enhanced allocation for education, imparting skills and healthcare – plays a significant role in fostering economic growth. One objective of the Eleventh Five Year Plan is to achieve good health for the people, especially the poor and the underprivileged. In order to do this, a comprehensive approach is needed that encompasses individual healthcare, public health, sanitation, clean drinking water, access to food, knowledge of hygiene and feeding practices. The Plan sought to facilitate convergence and development of public health systems and services that were responsive to health needs and aspirations of people. Importance was to be given to reducing disparities in health across regions and communities by ensuring access to affordable healthcare. It was, therefore, in the fitness of things that the Eleventh Five Year Plan, whose central theme was 'inclusive growth', substantially stepped up the allocation for health. The Plan document presented a well-conceived, comprehensive programme for the sector. According to the Prime Minister, the aim was to provide broad-based healthcare in rural areas through the NRHM.[62]

The key features of the Eleventh Five Year Plan are as follows:[63]

- 1.75 lakh sub-centres each with two ANMs at one sub-centre for each panchayat (five or six villages).
- 30,000 PHCs, one for a group of four or five sub-centres. Each PHC to have one lady health visitor and three staff nurses. There would also be an Ayurveda, Yoga and Naturopathy, Unani, Siddha and Homeopathy (AYUSH) physician.
- 1800 taluk or sub-divisional hospitals and 600 district hospitals to be fully equipped to provide quality health service.
- Enormous increase in the number of medical graduates, postgraduates and nurses needed to operate the system.
- Special attention was to be given to the health of marginalized groups like adolescent girls, women of all ages, children below the age of three, older persons, disabled and primitive tribal groups. It viewed gender as the cross-cutting theme across all schemes.

The Government of India drafted the National Health Bill[64] in 2009, by advising the legal framework to recognize the 'Right to Health' and 'Right to Healthcare' with a stated recognition to address the underlying social determinants of health. It was a bill to provide for protection and fulfilment of rights in relation to health and well-being, health equity and justice, including those related to all the underlying determinants of health as well as healthcare and for achieving the goal of health for all and for matters connected therewith or incidental thereto.[65] The Constitution of India, under Articles 14, 15 and 21, recognizes the Right to Life as a fundamental right and places obligations on the government to ensure protection and fulfilment of the Right to Health for all, without any inequality or discrimination. The Bill was divided into eight chapters, which distinctly stated the following: obligation of the government in relation to health, collective and individual rights in relation to health, implementation and monitoring mechanism, redressal mechanism for health rights and residuary offences, penalties and immunities.

A heartening point was that the Bill guaranteed that no person shall be denied care under any circumstances, including the inability to pay the requisite fees or charges. Prompt and necessary emergency medical treatment and critical care must be given by the healthcare provider concerned, including private providers.

As per the Bill, the healthcare provider, including the clinician, would be obligated to provide all information to the patients regarding the proposed treatment (risks, benefits, costs, etc.) and any alternative treatments that may be available for the particular condition/disease. There was a clause in the Bill that demanded that the user (i.e., the patient) respect the rights of the healthcare providers by treating them with respect, courtesy and dignity and refrain from any abuse or violent or abusive behaviour towards them or to the rights provided to them. The Bill envisaged the establishment of national- and state-level public health boards to formulate national policies on health, review strategies and ensure minimum standards for food, water, sanitation and housing. These boards would also lay down minimum standards and draw up protocols, norms and guidelines for diverse aspects of healthcare and treatment. The Bill provided for elaborate mechanisms for monitoring at the government and community levels.[66]

The preamble of the Bill is impressive to the extent that it promises 'protection and fulfillment of rights in relation to health and well-being, health equity and justice, including those related to all the underlying determinants of health and health care'. It grants that health is a fundamental human right that requires an overarching legal framework for providing essential public health services and functions, including powers to respond to public health emergencies, and also a common set of standards, norms and values. However, this is to facilitate the government's stewardship of the private health sector as a partner. It acknowledges the existing clauses regarding health in the Constitution and India's obligations as a signatory to several international treaties and agreements regarding Right to Health. Although all this sounds wonderful, it never acquires teeth as no rules are drawn to punish non-implementation of welfare services. These basic problems are rooted in the very definitions that the draft proposes or omits.[67]

Imrana Qadeer has pointed out the government's real intention behind this Bill. Explicit definitions of terms were neglected by the Bill making multiple legal interpretations possible. For example, it used terms such as the essential public health system, essential health facilities and healthcare services but did not make explicit their boundaries or which of these would be universal. The understanding of universal access was monetary – financial support for approaching a provider, public or private – affordable for the state, not actual services. While certain key social determinants were a part of the core responsibility of the state (safe drinking water, housing, sanitation, food), neither minimum standards to be achieved for these were spelled out nor were specific mechanisms set up to ensure inter-ministerial convergence.[68]

The Bill was more concerned with the private providers and did not specify the responsibility of the public sector except for its role in public health services for the marginalized. The issue of universalization therefore remained vague and devoid of a time plan. By putting the private and public providers in the same basket of an integrated system, the Bill ignored not only the basic contradictions of the two but also tilted the balance in favour of profits for the private sector by ensuring payments for services by the state without articulating shared objectives or conditions and liabilities of this partnership. The Bill proposed state- and district-level public health boards to implement obligation, evolve rules and regulations for recruitment from the open market, develop mechanisms for PPP and empower decentralized monitoring committees, but no principles for this implementation or regulation were articulated. No institutional redressal mechanisms for non-medical services like drinking water, sanitation, etc. were mentioned nor schedules, by-laws and rules were circulated. In other words, the Bill remained a policy document of the steward – the agency in service of rather than a law – for the private sector.[69]

Following the Bill, the Twelfth Five Year Plan Approach Paper, apparently oblivious of the financial cutbacks on the public sector in health and the ensuing loss of its pride and prestige, lamented about the sector's lack of capacity to deliver services. Ignoring failures to contain malaria, tuberculosis, leprosy and filariasis, it proposed expansion into new areas like handling deafness, care of the elderly, oral fluorosis, mental diseases, cancer, etc. It limited prevention to education and counselling, ignoring the conditions of poverty. While it proposed participation and community-based validation for the primary-level services, not a thought was spared for the regulation of tertiary institutions of the private sector that are at the core of the business of medical tourism. Promising more resources, insurance system, training and expansion of health manpower and drugs, the approach paper accepted that publicly financed healthcare does not necessarily mean provisioning of services. It emphasized the virtues of public–private partnerships, publicly financed insurance schemes such as RSBY, of outsourcing diagnostics and of a universal healthcare system on the same lines[70]

In 2009, when the Congress-led United Progressive Alliance (UPA) was back in power, India's growth rate was 9 per cent. Rajiv Arogyasree[71] and RSBY helped Congress for its success even after Left parties had left the UPA. The NRHM and its concept of the state's dominant role in healthcare and public provisioning of health services slid in importance. Instead, the Congress manifesto talked about expanding health insurance. The popularity of Rajiv Arogyasree and RSBY programmes increased the role of co-opting private healthcare sectors and this was very important for the policymakers, especially to the Planning Commission. The fact that Universal Health Coverage (UHC) was a political issue that could entail significant political dividends was also recognized.[72]

Before discussing the genesis and implementation of UHC and the subsequent report of the High-Level Expert Group (HLEG), a brief history of UHC should be dealt with. UHC is not a new concept in the domain of healthcare. It began to evolve in the nineteenth century when reforms were introduced in Germany by Bismarck.[73] The Beveridge Report (1942) ushered in British reforms in the 1940s leading to the introduction of the National Health Service (NHS) by Aneurin Bevan in 1948.[74] Since then, universal access to affordable healthcare has become a widely shared aspiration across the globe and over the last decade many low- and middle-income countries have adopted this approach in different models. The World Health Report[75] also endorsed this global movement.

The World Health Assembly adopted the term 'Universal Health Coverage' in 2005 and it has become the most widely used phrase in the global discourse on access and affordability of health services. WHO defines UHC as a 'state of health system performance, when all people receive the quality health services they need without suffering financial hardship'.[76]

In India, UHC entered the policy dialogue through the Public Health Foundation of India (PHFI), an initiative of the McKinsey consulting company. PHFI, chaired by a corporate honcho, was set up with a corpus of Rs 65 billion from the Indian Government, Rs 65 billion from the Bill and Melinda Gates Foundation and about Rs 4 billion of contribution promised by other corporate leaders.[77] It was a partnership between the government and the private sector and emerged as a think tank and became a one-stop solution for all donor- and foreign-funded research, including multinational pharmaceutical companies in the country. Contracted to come up with a plan to advocate UHC, PHFI was provided handsome grants from The Rockefeller Foundation in 2009 and flagged UHC as a global priority. UHC was the flavour of the season and the intention was to include it in the forthcoming Twelfth Five Year Plan.[78]

The Planning Commission was impatient at the performance of the NRHM and constituted the HLEG (chaired by Srinath Reddy, cardiologist and President of PHFI, India) on UHC in October 2010, with the mandate of developing a framework for providing easily accessible and affordable healthcare to all Indians. While financial protection was the principal objective of this initiative, it was recognized that the delivery of UHC also required the availability of adequate healthcare infrastructure, skilled health workforce and access to affordable drugs and technologies to ensure the entitled level and quality of care given to every citizen.[79]

Furthermore, the design and delivery of health programmes and services call for efficient management systems as well as active engagement of empowered communities. The original terms of reference directed the HLEG to address all of these needs of UHC. Since the social determinants of health have a profound influence not only on the health of populations but also on the ability of individuals to access healthcare, the HLEG decided to include a clear reference to them, though such determinants were conventionally regarded as falling in the domain of non-health sectors.

The HLEG undertook a situational analysis of each of the key elements of the existing health system and developed recommendations for reconfiguring and strengthening the health system to align it with the objectives of UHC, bridging the presently identified gaps and meeting the projected health needs of the people of India over the next decade. The Prime Minister declared, in his Independence Day address on 15 August 2011, that health would be accorded the highest priority in the Twelfth Five Year Plan (to be considered as 'health plan'), which would become operational in 2012.

The HLEG's vision of UHC transcended the narrow, inadequate and often inequitable view of UHC as merely a system of health insurance. UHC, in its understanding, moved beyond 'insurance' by providing an 'assurance' of healthcare for multiple needs and included health beyond healthcare, going beyond a mere illness response. UHC should address health in all of its dimensions and emphasize prevention and primary healthcare, which are ignored, neglected or even undermined by the usual systems of health insurance. Such an assurance has to be provided by the government, which has to act as the guarantor of UHC and ensure its success and sustainability, by mobilizing all societal resources and advance multi-sectoral actions. In this perspective, UHC is linked firmly to the Right to Health and converts an aspirational goal into an entitled provision. The HLEG also recognized that for such a vision of UHC to be realized a tax-based system of health financing was essential. This is also the global experience, wherein countries which have introduced UHC have mostly depended on general revenues rather than on unsteady streams of contributory health insurance, which offer incomplete coverage and restricted services. For UHC to succeed in India, political and financial commitments are required from the central as well as state governments.[80]

Ten principles have guided the formulation of the HLEG recommendations for introducing a system of UHC in India: (i) universality, (ii) equity, (iii) non-exclusion and non-discrimination, (iv) comprehensive care that is rational and of good quality, (v) financial protection, (vi) protection of patients' rights that guarantee appropriateness of care, patient choice, portability and continuity of care, (vii) consolidated and strengthened public health provisioning, (viii) accountability and transparency, (ix) community participation and (x) putting health in people's hands.

The HLEG recommendations were drawn from global best practices and lessons provided by Indian experience. The functioning of health systems in states like Tamil Nadu and Kerala was valuable in identifying the essential ingredients of a UHC framework. The experience of RSBY and various state-sponsored health insurance schemes for financial protection delivered inadequate results or had an unacceptable opportunity cost in neglected primary health services.[81] The Planning Commission incorporated some of the HLEG recommendations in its Twelfth Five Year Plan.[82]

The HLEG upheld the principle of universality, equity and higher investments in the health sector. It was clear that the state must be 'primarily and principally responsible for universal healthcare, which is an entitlement to comprehensive health security'. Hence, public sector services must be strengthened, improved and brought centre stage to ensure 'access and services' to all sections of the people. It recommended that user fees in public institutions should be discontinued and participation of citizens must go beyond existing forms of community involvement in pre-conceived programmes of provisioning and monitoring healthcare. It was argued that UHC could succeed only if it was founded on common interests of all sections, 'social solidarity and cross-subsidization across classes'. Hence, it proposed a single universal method of financing through general and differential health taxation and recommended that '70 per cent of it should go to primary healthcare'.[83]

If India has to improve outcomes and equity in access, increasing public health expenditure will be critical. It will have to reverse the post-1991 declining trends in public health spending and move towards the UPA government's target of allocating 3 per cent of the GDP as public health expenditure.[84]

The Twelfth Plan based on the HLEG report made a reasonable effort at assessment of the current health scenario and suggested a strategy that would entail a substantial increase in public health spending from 1.04 per cent of GDP at the end of the Eleventh Plan to 1.87 per cent by the end of the Twelfth Plan, the expansion of RSBY, expansion of medical education, access to free medicines in public facilities, regulation of the private healthcare sector, contracting in private services where public facilities were deficient and so on.[85]

There was no clarity on the nature of health financing with regard to creation of a single-payer system from the welter of government-funded social insurance schemes. The role of the private sector was emphasized without caveats on the nature of contracting, accountability and regulation. While integrated care was mentioned, no pathway was indicated for the continuum of care across primary, secondary and tertiary services across the maze of India's mixed health system[86] (see Table 2.1).

Table 2.1 Health Expenditure Trends in India

Year	Total Public Health Expenditure (Rs. Billions)	Per Cent of GDP	Private Health Expenditure (Rs. Billions)	Per Cent of GDP	Per Cent Private to Total Health Expenditure
1993–1991	76.81	0.98	195.43	2.50	71.78
1994–1995	85.65	0.93	278.59	3.04	76.48
1995–1996	96.01	0.89	329.23	3.07	77.42
1996–1997	109.35	0.88	373.41	3.000	77.35
1997–1998	127.21	0.92	458.99	3.30	78.30
1998–1999	151.13	0.94	653.40	4.04	81.21
1999–2000	172.16	0.96	835.17	4.76	82.91
2000–2001	186.13	0.98	981.68	5.18	84.06
2001–2002	194.54	0.94	1,100.00	5.32	84.90
2002–2003	197.32	0.88	1,250.00	5.60	86.36
2004–2005	258	0.85	1,529*	5	86.82
2006–2007	365	0.91	1,854*	5.8	85.19
2007–2008	431	0.90	2,042*	5.1	84.78
2008–2009	519	0.97	2,249*	4.24	81.25
2009–2010	606	0.99	2,477*	4.05	80.34
2010–2011	716	0.98	2,730*	3.76	79.22
2011–2012	929	1.04	3,007*	3.42	76.40
2012–2013	997	0.99	3,312*	3.29	76.86
2013–2014	1219	1.06	3,600**	3.13	74.70
2014–2015	1498RE+	1.15	4,000**	3.08	72.75
2015–2016	1570BE+	1.05	4,500**	3.00	74.13

Source Public: Finance Accounts of Central and State Governments up to 2011–2012 and RBI's Finances of State Governments, and Union Budget Expenditure Statements for subsequent years; Private: CSO-GOI – Private Final Consumption Expenditures, National Accounts Statistics 2003 (1993–1994 Series).

*Since the available Private Finance Consumption Expenditure (PFCE) Data beyond 2003–2004 is only available based on 2004–2005 series and non-comparable, the estimates have been calculated by the author for private expenditures based on the ratio difference of PFCE between 1993–1994 and 2004–2005 series, for example, for 2002–2003 the 1993–1994 series was 1.6 times the 2004–2005 series – overall this appears to be an underestimate for private health expenditure.
** author estimate
*RE = revised estimate.
*BE = budget estimate.[87]

It is quite evident from the data that public finance of healthcare is weakening and private expenditure is growing. This needs to be changed if India has to move towards Universal Access to Health. Apart from raising the budgetary commitments, there would be need for critical structural changes in the way resources were allocated, budgets planned, service delivery organized, the way public health institutions were governed and so on.[88]

Instead of an integrated health service with primary healthcare getting support from the secondary and tertiary, the thrust of the planning process had been to fragment health service into independent components – UHC, tertiary care and NRHM – in the name of providing rural and urban health services. In each of these strategies, PPPs, commercialization and appropriation of the public resources were the dominant trends. UHC thus no more remained the state-led integrated and inclusive service but became a 'Trojan horse of the neoliberal strategy'. The HLEG report stuck to fertility control programmes based on technology and failed to locate fertility within the same social determinants that cause ill health. Similarly, it continued to mistake primary-level healthcare for comprehensive primary healthcare, dazzled with high-tech medical care and the norms of care set by corporate hospitals. The recommendations totally ignored the vast presence of traditional practitioners in the country and the fact that in 14 major states, about 20–98 per cent of households reported using them in the past three months and in five of these the use was 60–98 per cent. While health security is inclusive of a broad range of welfare services, these were left to overall planning without confronting the extent of non-availability of food, drinking water, housing and sanitation and its impact on health. By ignoring the constraint, these social determinants impose on achieving health through technology-based services, the group of experts remained confined to intra-systemic techno-managerial solutions giving them priority over social and structural issues. The committee essentially believed that the 'Health sector primarily focuses on the delivery of curative services'. It thereby ignored the history of the evolution of public health service in India that apart from using curative care for prevention built promotive programmes by provisioning food and food supplements and sanitation and drinking water to vulnerable populations. Except for the proposal of state public health acts and a system of providing free drugs for the Essential Health Package (EHP), not much was new. Strengthening of tertiary care was an independent task, and private sector facilities were put centre stage with the logic that they cater to 60 per cent of in-patients. Caught between the welfare approach of the HLEG report and the crass neoliberalism of the steering committee, the draft chapter on health in the Twelfth Plan attempted to find a middle path but could only make it less crass.[89]

Another crucial issue that needs mentioning is that the Fourteenth Finance Commission submitted its report adding a new twist to the already unhappy tale. As per the Constitution, it is the responsibility of the states to deliver health services. To help states overcome their fiscal incapacities, the central government provides financial resources under Centrally Sponsored Schemes (CSS) that have often been resisted by states as an 'encroachment' on their turf. To correct this vertical asymmetry, the Fourteenth Finance Commission increased the proportional share of the states under unconditional grants from 32 per cent to 42 per cent of the total amounts devolved to the states, thereby reducing the central government's space for making discretionary grants under the CSS mechanism. While the rationale for this strategic shift was to provide states with more fiscal space and flexibility to set their own priorities and spending preferences, the central government reacted by slashing budgets for several social sector schemes that impact health (HIV/AIDS and NRHM), primary education, water supply and nutrition. The central share was reduced from 75 per cent to 60 per cent, burdening the state further.[90]

Mention should be made that for the first time a Plan document talked of universal healthcare, albeit in a limited way, but the process was aborted with the three member-NITI Aayog (which replaced the Planning Commission) rejecting the HLEG as well as the diluted Twelfth Plan health strategy and pushing for a rapid expansion of health insurance and enhanced the role of the private sector.[91]

The debates and arguments between the Planning Commission and the health ministry basically reflected two viewpoints. One viewpoint believes in strengthening and investing in the public sector, using the private sector to supplement its effort, and the other advocated by NITI Aayog sought to privatize the healthcare sector and sustain it through a web of financing mechanisms and subsidies.[92]

Between these two views, the HLEG ought to have found in the government its natural ally. It unintendedly undermined the NRHM that, given all the constraints and problems, had been so impressively rolled out in the states. The harsh truth is that India has supply constraints in terms of the availability of doctors, paramedics, other supporting infrastructure and resources.[93]

It was against this backdrop of confusion that there was a change of government. In 2014, BJP came to power. RSBY was shifted to the health ministry without its budget for good measure. Dissociated with the health ministry, RSBY had undermined the efforts being made by NRHM in strengthening the functioning and quality of care delivered in public hospitals. By accrediting all and sundry private hospitals with a disregard for the quality or standards, the impact was weakened in terms of reducing the OOP expenditure.[94]

In the Twelfth Plan, the NRHM came to be known as NHM, consisting of four components the NRHM, the National Urban Health Mission (NUHM), disease control programmes and non-communicable diseases. Funds are no longer to be released to the state finance departments but routed through the state finance departments. Some new initiatives were launched in the budget of 2016 like the National Dialysis Programme (NDP) was introduced. Under this scheme, district hospitals were to be provided funding support to supply these services in a PPP mode. Customs duties were waived to facilitate the import of the required equipment.[95]

The Tenth and Eleventh Five Year Plans identified the huge inequalities in access to healthcare and also increasing the OOP expenditure. A new draft of National Health Policy 2015 was introduced for comments by the government in January 2015, and new hope for UHC arose. The draft NHP 2015 gave emphasis on equity, universality, inclusive partnerships, affordability, pluralism and accountability among its key principles.

NHP 2015 reviewed the urgent need to improve the performance of health systems. It was being formulated in the last year of the Millennium Declaration and its goals in the global context of all nations committed to moving towards Universal Health Coverage. Given the two-way linkage between economic growth and health status, this National Health Policy is a declaration of the determination of the government to leverage economic growth to achieve health outcomes. The policy will ensure universal access to affordable healthcare services in an assured mode – the promise of health assurance is an important catalyst for the framing of a new health policy.[96]

The new Policy document discussed that while there was considerable progress towards the Millennium Development Goals for maternal and child mortality as well as achievements of the NRHM, reduction in the burden of communicable diseases and big successes like the elimination of polio from India, there were many persisting challenges such as health services were quantitatively inadequate and their quality was often not known, low public expenditure on health and people often had to pay out of their pockets to avail health services at risk of falling into poverty, and the emerging burden of non-communicable diseases (NCDs). Fortunately, these challenges were being recognized and there were incremental steps and clearly articulated intentions to improve access to quality health services at a cost affordable to the people as a part of ongoing discourses on UHC in India. Non-communicable diseases were given importance in the draft NHP 2015.

As far as the question of financing and expenditure of the health sector is concerned, there was the progress to create a 'National Health Accounts' (NHA) for India, as well. The most recent NHA provides information for the years 2004–2005, published in the year 2009.[97]

While crediting the NRHM for several innovations, the NHP draft recognized that much emphasis was being given to select reproductive and child health services compared to national disease control programmes and also to a wider range of healthcare services. Social determinants of health were also ignored. The draft also admitted that primary care had been very selective, covering less than 20 per cent of the healthcare needs.

Although there was an increase in public financing on healthcare from 1.04 to 2.5 per cent of the GDP, the draft was diffident about achieving this because of fiscal straining. The policy stated that over 63 million persons were exposed to the threat of being rendered poor every year by unaffordable healthcare expenditure and recognized that financial protection was to be rendered to the poor as well as the non-poor vulnerable to such a threat.[98]

There was a bold declaration that the Right to Health would be provided with a legal framework through a National Health Right Act, which would ensure health as a fundamental right. The policy with respect to urban health would be to address the primary healthcare needs of the urban population. The NUHM would need to be strengthened and adequately financed to achieve this. NUHM would cover all state capitals, district headquarters and cities/towns with more than 50,000 populations. Within this primary care approach there would be a special focus on poor populations living in listed and unlisted slums, other vulnerable populations such as homeless, ragpickers, street children, rickshaw pullers, construction workers, sex workers and temporary migrants.[99]

Seven key policy shifts were highlighted in the draft NHP 2015:

1. In Primary Care: From selective care that was fragmented from secondary/ tertiary care to assured comprehensive care that had continuity with higher levels.
2. In Secondary and Tertiary Care: From an input-oriented, budget line financing to an output-based strategic purchasing.
3. In Public Hospitals: From user fees and cost recovery-based public hospitals to assured free drugs, diagnostic and emergency services to all in public health facilities.
4. In Infrastructure and Human Resource Development: From normative approaches in their development to targeted approaches to reach under-serviced areas.
5. In Urban Health: From token under-financed interventions to on-scale assured interventions that reach the urban poor and establish linkages with national programmes: scaling up of the interventions with a focus on the urban poor and achieving convergence among the wider determinants of health.
6. In National Health Programmes: Integration with health systems for effectiveness and contributing to strengthening health systems for efficiency.
7. In AYUSH services: From standalone AYUSH to a three-dimensional mainstreaming.

Engagement of non-physician service providers from different categories of allied health professionals, along with AYUSH professionals was proposed. It also proposed that the promotion of yoga in the work place, in the schools and in the community would also be an important form of health promotion that had a special appeal and acceptability in the Indian context.[100]

As the policy moved to address secondary and tertiary care, there was a growing need for dependence on private healthcare. Ambiguity regarding the role of the public sector is amplified when the draft says that the mindset must move away from regarding public sector healthcare as free but instead consider it as prepaid care. While this correctly holds the public sector accountable for quality, it does not say how will this happen if the health budget is not increased and the governance of the health system is not improved?[101]

The policy calls for all national and state health insurance schemes to be aligned into a single insurance scheme and a single fund pool reducing fragmentation. This is highly desirable and will transform the patchwork quilt of government-funded social insurance schemes into a single-payer safety net.

The Union Budget of 2015 had a clear disconnect with the draft health policy. While there was a marginal increase in the allocations to the health sector, in terms of GDP, the public finance in the Centre had fallen. The increase in tax exemption limits for medical insurance and medical reimbursement may provide some relief to the salaried class, but this too would be limited to what private health insurance and private hospitals would cover for some illnesses. This would exclude 90 per cent of the population from these limited benefits. Creating more All India Institutes of Medical Sciences, which provide tertiary care, as proposed in the Union Budget of 2014 and 2015, would not redress the neglect of primary and secondary care. Tax concessions on private health insurance premiums and provision for opting out of the ESI indicated that the government wished to provide the higher income groups and employees the private insurance route for purchase of healthcare from private providers.[102]

The previous UPA government had committed to raising the contribution of the public exchequer to health to up to 3 per cent of the GDP over the period of the implementation of the first phase of the National Rural Health Mission from 2005 to 2011, a promise that remained elusive. The Narendra Modi government, in its very first budget, presented in 2014, slashed the healthcare allocation by 20 per cent in one go, imperilling even the day-to-day activities of many disease control programmes. Furthermore, Arvind Panagariya, the vice-chairman of NITI Aayog, feels that the healthcare needs of all poor can well be taken care of in just about three-quarters of 1 per cent of the GDP (quoted in Kurian 2015). What is all the more intriguing is that the magnanimity of our rulers towards their countrymen seems to have dried up precisely at a time when they are making claims of India being the fastest-growing economy in the world. Nevertheless, though the odds remain onerous, one can always hope for a turnaround.[103]

In the fall of 2015, the headquarters of the United Nations in New York, amid celebrations of the seventieth anniversary of the organization, adopted a historic set of 17 goals and 169 targets called the Sustainable Development Goals (SDGs). Building upon the MDGs, these new sets of goals are directed to show the way forward. They are committed to achieving sustainable development of the civilization in three dimensions, i.e., economic, social and environmental, in a balanced and integrated manner. The SDGs are integrated and indivisible, global in nature and universally applicable. The governments world over are expected to set their own national policies containing their dedicated priorities, resources and targets, being guided by the SDGs yet keeping national circumstances in view.[104]

NHP 2017 built on the progress made since the last NHP 2002. The developments were captured in the document 'Backdrop to National Health Policy 2017 – Situation Analyses', Ministry of Health and Family Welfare, Government of India.[105]

The main goal for health in the Sustainable Development Goals is ensuring healthy lives and promoting well-being for all age groups. The first target is to reduce the 'MMR' to less than 70 per lakh live births. India has seen a decrease of three-quarters between 1990 and 2015. From the baseline of 556 in 1990, MMR had reduced to 162 per lack live births. The new policy of the country aimed at achieving a target of 100 by the year 2020. The policy sought to enhance provisions for reproductive morbidity, besides ensuring free, comprehensive primary care services for all aspects of reproductive maternal and child health. The policy intended to sustain antenatal coverage at 90 per cent and skilled attendance of birth at above 90 per cent.

The NHP intended to reduce the under-five mortality to 23, neonatal mortality to 16 and still birth to single-digit numbers. It assured complete immunization for more than 90 per cent of newborns.[106]

A target of this goal was to end the epidemics of HIV/TB/malaria, and neglected to combat tropical diseases and hepatitis, waterborne and other communicable diseases. The NHP had a target to achieve and maintain the cure rate of more than 85 per cent in new sputum-positive cases of TB and reach elimination by the year 2025. For HIV, the target of 90:90:90 was to be achieved by 2020. Achieving elimination of leprosy by 2018, kala azar by 2017 and lymphatic filariasis by 2017 was targeted.[107]

National Health Policy 2017 aimed at providing good quality healthcare services in an assured manner to all by addressing current and emerging challenges arising from the ever-changing socio-economic, epidemiological and technological scenarios. Among the key policy principles, equity, affordability, accountability, inclusive partnership and decentralization are worth mentioning. NHP-2017 also identified seven priority areas for improving the environment for health. These priority areas needing coordinated action included:[108]

1. The Swachh Bharat Abhiyan.
2. Balanced, healthy diets and regular exercises.
3. Addressing tobacco, alcohol and substance abuse.
4. Yatri Suraksha – preventing deaths due to rail and road traffic accidents.
5. Nirbhaya Nari – an action against gender violence.
6. Reduced stress and improved safety in the work place.
7. Reducing indoor and outdoor air pollution.

NHP 2017 faces the challenging task of ensuring affordable, quality medical care to every citizen of the nation. To achieve Universal Health Coverage by 2025, NHP 2017 assures comprehensive primary care to one and all. Both the quantifiable and measurable goals have been laid down. It has been proposed to set up health and wellness centres, which would provide a full range of preventive and promotive services to prevent diseases and enhance well-being. To make this a reality, every family would have a health card that links them to a primary care facility and be eligible for a defined package of services anywhere in the country. The policy recommends that health centres be established on geographical norms apart from population norms. To provide comprehensive care, the policy recommends a matching human resource development strategy, effective logistics support system and referral backup. This would also necessitate upgradation of the existing sub-centres and reorienting PHCs to provide a comprehensive set of preventive, promotive, curative and rehabilitative services. It would entail providing access to assured AYUSH healthcare services, as well as support documentation and validation of local home and community-based practices. The policy also advocates the research and validation of tribal medicines. Leveraging the potential of digital health for two-way systemic linkages between the various levels of care, viz., primary, secondary and tertiary, would ensure continuity of care. To address the serious shortage of human resources, the policy has proposed: (i) reviving the multipurpose male worker cadre, (ii) empowerment of ASHAs to undertake preventive education at the community level and (iii) training AYUSH doctors, nurses and paramedics for six months on public health so as to position them in the health and wellness centres. From the current spending of 1.15 per cent on public health, the policy envisages raising the spending to 2.5 per cent of GDP by 2025.[109]

Free primary care provision by the public sector, supplemented by the strategic purchase of secondary care hospitalization and tertiary care services from both public and non-government sectors to fill critical gaps, would be the main strategy of assuring healthcare services. The policy envisages the strategic purchase of secondary and tertiary care services as a short-term measure. Strategic purchasing refers to the government acting as a single payer.[110] Collaboration can also be done for certain services where a team of specialized human resources and domain-specific organizational experience is required. Private providers, especially those working in rural and remote areas or with under-serviced communities, could be offered encouragement through the provision of appropriate skills to meet public health goals, opportunities for skill upgradation to serve the community better, participation in disease notification and surveillance efforts, as well as sharing and supporting certain high-value services. In order to provide access and financial protection at secondary and tertiary care levels, the policy proposes free drugs, free diagnostics and free emergency care services in all public hospitals. To address the growing challenges of urban health, the policy advocates scaling up the National Urban Health Mission to cover the entire urban population within the next five years with sustained financing.[111]

Public hospitals have to be viewed as part of the tax-financed single-payer healthcare system, where the care is prepaid and cost-efficient. This outlook implies that quality of care would be imperative, and the public hospitals and facilities would undergo periodic measurements and certification of the level of quality. The policy endorses that the public hospitals would provide universal access to a progressively wide array of free drugs and diagnostics with a suitable leeway to the states to suit their context. The policy seeks to eliminate the risks of inappropriate treatment by maintaining adequate standards of diagnosis and treatment. The policy recognizes the need for an information system with comprehensive data on the availability and utilization of services not only in public hospitals but also in non-government sector hospitals. State public health systems should be able to provide all emergency health services other than services covered under national health programmes.[112]

The policy affirms that the tertiary care services are best organized along the lines of regional, zonal and apex referral centres. It recommends that the government should set up new medical colleges, nursing institutions and AIIMS in the country following this broad principle. Regional disparities in the distribution of these institutions must be addressed. The policy supports periodic review and standardization of the fee structure and quality of clinical training in the private sector medical colleges.[113]

The policy recognizes the inter-relationship between communicable disease control programmes and public health system strengthening. For the Integrated Disease Surveillance Programme, the policy advocates the need for districts to respond to the communicable disease priorities of their locality. The policy recognizes the need to halt and reverse the growing incidence of chronic diseases. It recommends setting up a National Institute of Chronic Diseases, including trauma, to generate evidence for adopting cost-effective approaches and to showcase best practices. This policy will support an integrated approach where screening for the most prevalent NCDs with secondary prevention would make a significant impact on the reduction of morbidity and preventable mortality. This would be incorporated into the comprehensive primary healthcare network with linkages to specialist consultations and follow-up at the primary level. Emphasis on medication and access for select chronic illnesses on a round-the-year basis would be ensured. Screening for oral, breast and cervical cancer and for chronic obstructive pulmonary disease (COPD) will be focused on in addition to hypertension and diabetes. The policy focus is also on research. It emphasizes developing a protocol for mainstreaming AYUSH as integrated medical care. This has a huge potential for effective prevention and therapy that is safe and cost-effective.[114]

The existing government-financed health insurance schemes shall be aligned to cover the selected benefit package of secondary and tertiary care services purchased from public, not-for-profit and private sectors in the same order of preference, subject to the availability of quality services on time as per the defined norms. The policy recommends creating a robust independent mechanism to ensure adherence to standard treatment protocols by public and non-government hospitals. In this context the policy recognizes the need for mandatory disclosure of treatment and success rates across facilities in a transparent manner. It recommends compliance with the right of patients to access information about their condition and treatment. For need-based purchasing of secondary and tertiary care from non-government sectors, multi-stakeholder institutional mechanisms would be created at the Centre and State levels – in the forms of trusts or registered societies with institutional autonomy.[115]

Although NHP 2017 provided a road map for future development in the healthcare sector, there were certain challenges and contradictions. Considering the budget allocation made by the Government of India for the health sector, the targets mentioned in the NHP seem overambitious. The expenditure on health in India is one of the lowest in the world at 1.4 per cent of the GDP. NHP 2017 aims to increase this to about 2.5 per cent, which again is much less than the required 5–6 per cent. The money allocated for health in the Union Budget 2017 was nowhere near to achieving the target of even 2.5 per cent. Public investment in primary care is barely $17 per capita, whereas estimates prepared for Sustainable Developmental Goal 3's target of Universal Health Coverage to essential care by 2030 is about $85 per capita. The low spending on public health has resulted in poorly developed primary healthcare infrastructure, and even if available, it largely remains underutilized like providing only 15 per cent of the services to the under-five children. The non-availability of skilled human resources and essential infrastructure is a serious barrier as more than two-thirds of this deficit is in the 'underserved' areas that have only a fifth of the money and three-quarters of the disease burden.

Another concern is regarding the primary care services, which the policy states would be provided by the government. The policy assumes that the public and private sectors can function and compete in the same space, thereby simplifying the complete dynamics. NHP 2017 time and again mentions 'strategic purchasing' of private services for filling the so-called gap to address the issue of 'supply side' imbalances. But in reality, this gap is huge, as the private sector is providing about 70 per cent of out-patients department (OPD) and 60 per cent of in-patient care, especially at the secondary and tertiary levels. In this context, public hospitals provide a rational and cheaper care and thus keep a check on the private sector from unnecessary procedures leading to profiteering. It would then be pertinent to invest in public hospitals in the first instance before pushing to purchase services from the private sector. The next concern is the weak commitment made to building the required infrastructure in urban and rural areas for delivering primary healthcare services. NHP 2017 affirms the desire to achieve the IPHS but fails to assess its fiscal implications.[116]

The primary healthcare system in India has evolved since its Independence, and there is an elaborate network of nearly 200,000 Government Primary Healthcare Facilities (GPHCFs), both in rural and urban areas. The existing GPHCFs deliver a narrow range of services, due to a variety of reasons including, at times, the non-availability of providers as well. Thus, the GPHCFs in India are grossly underutilized, and excluding the mother and child health services, in 2013–2014, only 11.5 per cent of rural and 3.9 per cent of urban people in need of health services used this vast network. People in India either choose a higher level of government facilities for primary healthcare needs (which results in an issue of subsidiarity) or attend a private provider (which results in the OOP expenditure); both situations are not good for a well-functioning health system. The challenges of weak PHC in India are increasingly being recognized and acknowledged. NHP 2017 proposed to strengthen PHC systems and invest two-thirds or more government health spending on PHC, with an increase in overall government funding for health. Following NHP 2017, the Government of India announced the Ayushman Bharat Programme (ABP) in February 2018 to achieve the vision of Universal Health Coverage with two components:

(a) Health and Wellness Centres (HWCs) to strengthen and deliver Comprehensive Primary Healthcare (CPHC) services for the entire population.
(b) Pradhan Mantri Jan Arogya Yojana.

This initiative has been designed to meet the SDGs and their underlining commitment, which is to 'leave no one behind'.[117] It is an attempt to move from the sectoral and segmented approach of health service delivery to a comprehensive need-based healthcare service. This scheme aims at undertaking path-breaking interventions to holistically address the healthcare system (covering prevention, promotion and ambulatory care) at the primary, secondary and tertiary levels.

In February 2018, the Government of India announced the creation of 150,000 HWCs by transforming the existing sub-centres and primary health centres. The first HWC was launched on 14 April 2018, and by 31 March 2020, a total of 38,595 Ayushman Bharat HWCs (AB-HWCs) were operational across India. Currently, the SCs and PHCs meet only 20 per cent of healthcare needs and provide services limited to reproductive, maternal, newborn, child and adolescent health (RMNCH+A) and some communicable disease management. Under the HWC initiative, these sub-centres and primary health centres will be upgraded to handle NCDs like cancer, cardio-vascular disease (CVD), diabetes and respiratory diseases, mental illnesses and other chronic diseases, as these are currently the major cause of mortality and morbidity due to the epidemiological transition. These HWCs will provide a wider range of free drugs and diagnostics, services related to elderly care, oral health, ear, nose and throat (ENT) care, eye care and basic emergency care, in addition to the RMNCH+A and basic infection care.

HWCs are envisaged to deliver an expanded range of services to address the primary healthcare needs of the entire population in their area, expanding access, universality and equity close to the community. The emphasis on health promotion and prevention is designed to bring focus on keeping people healthy by engaging and empowering individuals and communities to choose healthy behaviours and make changes that reduce the risk of developing chronic diseases and morbidities.

There is a global consensus that Universal Health Coverage can only be achieved on the foundation of a stronger primary healthcare system. There is renewed attention on strengthening and delivering comprehensive primary healthcare services in India through HWCs. While the AB-HWCs aim to address the existing challenges in the PHC system, the effectiveness and success will be dependent upon a rapid transition from policy to the implementation stage, focus on both supply- and demand-side interventions, engagement of community and civil society and other stakeholders, focus on effective and functional referral linkages, ongoing learnings, innovations and mid-course corrections, effective linkage and coordination between two the components of ABP, additional and complementary initiatives by the states, sustained political will and monitoring and evaluation of the process, among others.[118]

The second component under Ayushman Bharat is the Pradhan Mantri Jan Arogya Yojana or PM-JAY as it is popularly known. This scheme was launched on 23 September 2018 in Ranchi, Jharkhand, by Prime Minister Narendra Modi.

PM-JAY is the largest health assurance scheme in the world, which aims at providing a health cover of Rs 5 lakh per family per year for secondary and tertiary care hospitalization to over 10.74 crore poor and vulnerable families (approximately 50 crore beneficiaries) that form the bottom 40 per cent of the Indian population. The households included are based on the deprivation and occupational criteria of Socio-Economic Caste Census 2011 (SECC 2011) for rural and urban areas, respectively. PM-JAY was earlier known as the National Health Protection

Scheme (NHPS). It subsumed the then-existing RSBY, which had been launched in 2008 and also the Senior Citizen Health Insurance Scheme. The coverage mentioned under PM-JAY, therefore, also includes families that were covered in RSBY but are not present in the SECC 2011 database. PM-JAY is fully funded by the government, and the cost of implementation is shared between the central and state governments.[119]

The government is 'steadily but surely progressing towards the goal of Universal Health Coverage'. This mega healthcare project, named 'Modicare' or 'Namocare' (by Union Home Minister Amit Shah) indeed promises to provide secondary and tertiary care hospitalization and covers both prevention and health promotion.

Theoretically, the scheme will target up to 500 million individuals from financially vulnerable households that accounts for 41.3 per cent of the population, according to Census data. Under the NHPS, four in ten Indians can avail of secondary and tertiary care in government and private hospitals within the insurance cap earmarked per family. A new national health agency will be instituted under the scheme to oversee its implementation at the state level. The identification of beneficiaries is to be done by consulting the SECC 2011.[120]

RSBY, which was the precursor to Modicare, was targeted at BPL families and has been implemented in 15 states. NHPS was, in fact, announced in the 2016 Budget – the only difference being that the sum assured was raised from Rs 30,000 to Rs 1.5 lakh then and to Rs 5 lakh later. The scheme has not been operationalized in the last two years. Moreover, not even 50 per cent of the funds under the existing health cover scheme have been spent in the past year. Many large states already have better designed insurance schemes in place. Moreover, a hike in budgetary allocation for health was less in 2018 as compared to 2017. When in 2017, the budgetary allocation to the health sector was raised to 28%, the country hailed the move. It was the first time when health was given much-needed attention. India's health budget had not changed much since 2009 and remained merely between 0.98% and 1.18% of the GDP, one of the lowest in the world. Although the Narendra Modi government did reveal its plan of increasing healthcare spending by 2.5% by 2025, the lower increase in 2018 deviated from the roadmap. But the National Health Mission – the flagship scheme – has also seen a decrease in allocation. While Rs 30,801.56 crore was spent on NHM in 2017–2018, in 2018–2019, the allocation was Rs 30,129.61 crore.

The current free healthcare plan is far bigger than its predecessors. Now, the most pertinent question is, how exactly will the government find the resources to implement this scheme? Former Union Finance Minister Arun Jaitley requested the private companies and corporate bodies to support the government's initiatives through corporate social responsibility (CSR) activities.[121]

NHPS, which is modelled along the lines of Obamacare, indicates the government's intent to further the beneficiary pool for healthcare standard operating procedures (SOPs). One of the main reasons Obamacare was controversial was the 'individual mandate', a provision that allowed the government to raise funds by penalizing people who did not have health insurance. Other modes of revenue generation for the healthcare policy included cuts in government funding, increasing taxes on high-income individuals and a variety of annual fees and surcharges.

But perhaps the biggest unique selling proposition (USP) of Obamacare was that insurance companies could not turn down or overcharge people with pre-existing medical conditions.

Modicare, as it stands now, is geared more towards taking care of the corporate healthcare industry's interests in the name of the poor.

It is actually insurance of insurance companies.

The discussion of several healthcare policies, plans and programmes from the time of Independence reveals that none of the governments at the Centre has given serious attention to the health issues of this vastly populated nation. It was not the inability that stood as the hindrance but the will to restructure the healthcare services. Proposals were made in several policies but the issue of implementing them to reduce inequity was not seriously addressed. The changing profile of diseases prepared the ground for the techno-centric and insurance-based approach to healthcare. The primary healthcare sector, which needed more attention for addressing the health problems of the rural masses was ignored. On the contrary, policies of healthcare tried to strengthen the tertiary and secondary level healthcare sectors.

Notes

1 Planning Commission, Government of India, *Eighth Five Year Plan Highlights* (New Delhi: Directorate of Advertising and Visual Publicity, Government of India, 1992).
2 Rao, *Do We Care?*, 17.
3 For details of private healthcare developments in India in the pre-liberalisation era see Sunil Nandaraj, "Beyond Law and the Lord: Quality of Private Health Quality", *Economic and Political Weekly* 29, no. 27 (January 1994): 1680–85.
4 Purendra Prasad, "Health Care Reforms: Do They Ensure Social Protection for the Labouring Poor?", in *Equity and Access: Health Care Studies in India*, ed. Purendra Prasad and Amar Jessani (New Delhi: OUP, 2018) (Hereafter cited as Prasad, "Health Care Reforms").
5 Rao, *Do We Care?*, 16. Also see Sunil Nandaraj, "Unregulated and Unaccountable: Private Health Providers", *Economic and Political Weekly* 42, no. 04 (January 2012): 12.
6 Mukhopadhyay, *Report of the Independent Commission*, 40.
7 Ibid.
8 Rao, op. cit., 17.
9 Mukhopadhyay, *Report of the Independent Commission*, 41.
10 Ibid., 41.
11 Ibid.
12 Rao, op. cit., 18.
13 Mukhopadhyay, *Report of the Independent Commission*, 40.
14 Rao, op cit., 21–22. Also see Mukhopadhyay, *Report of the Independent Commission*.
15 Mukhopadhyay, *Report of the Independent Commission*, 40.
16 For details on user fees, see World Bank Documents (See 1985, 1987, 1993, 1997) Bijoya Roy and Siddharta Gupta, "Public-Private Partnership and User Fees in Healthcare: Evidence from West Bengal", *Economic and Political Weekly* xlvi, no. 38 (September 2011). Mylene Lagardea and Natasha Palmer, "The Impact of User Fees on Health Service Utilization in Low- and Middle-Income Countries: How Strong is the Evidence", *Bulletin of the World Health Organization* 86 (2008): 839–48; West

Bengal Health Policy Note, *World Bank South Asia Region,* June 2004, Oommen C. Kurian Suchitra, and Wagle Prashant Raymus, *Mapping the Flow of User Fees in a Public Hospital* (Bombay: Centre for Enquiry into Health and Allied Themes, 2011); Amrita Bagchi, "Reforms or Dictates: The Role of the Donor Agencies on Health Care in West Bengal", *Global South –Sephis e-magazine* 7, no. 3 (July 2011).

17 Rao, op. cit., 18. Also see Rama Baru, "Commercialisation and the Poverty of Public Health Services in India", in *Public Health and Private Wealth: Stem Cells, Surrogates and Other Strategic Bodies,* ed. Sarah Hodges and Mohan Rao (New Delhi: Oxford University Press, 2016).

18 Rama V. Baru and Madhurima Nundy, "Blurring of Boundaries: Public-Private Partnerships in Health Services in India", *Economic and Political Weekly* 43, no. 4 (January–February 2008): 63. (Hereafter cited as Baru and Nundy, "Blurring of Boundaries"). Also see Rao, *Do We Care?*; Bijoya Roy and Siddharta Gupta, "Public-Private Partnership and User Fees in Healthcare: Evidence from West Bengal", *Economic and Political Weekly* xlvi, no. 38 (September 2011), https://www.epw.in /journal/2021/36/perspectives/public-private-partnerships-healthcare.html, accessed on 20.11.2021; "Financing and Delivery of Health Care Services in India", *National Commission on Macroeconomics and Health, Background Paper,* Ministry of Health & Family Welfare, Government of India (New Delhi: August, 2005).

19 Duggal, "Historical Review of Health Policy Making", 38.

20 Ibid.

21 Baru and Nundy, "Blurring of Boundaries", 63.

22 World Bank, *World Development Report 1993: Investing in Health* (New York: Oxford University Press, 1993).

23 M. Fisk, "Neoliberalism and the Slow Death of Public Healthcare in Mexico", *Journal of Socialism and Democracy* 14, no. 1 (2000): 63–84, cited in Shailendra Hooda, "Health System in Transition in India: Journey from State Provisioning to Privatization", *World Review of Political Economy* 11, no. 4 (Winter 2020): 506–32.

24 World Bank, *"India: Raising the Sights: Better Health Systems for India's Poor." World Bank Report no. 22304* (Washington, DC: World Bank, 2001).

25 Prasad, "Health Care Reforms", 52. Also see Imrana Qadeer, Kasturi Sen and K.R. Nayar, ed. *Public Health and Poverty of Reforms* (New Delhi: Sage Publications, 2001).

26 Duggal, "Historical Review of Health Policy Making", 38.

27 GOI, *National Health Policy-2002.* Department of Health, Ministry of Health and Family Welfare (New Delhi: Government of India, 2002a).

28 Ibid.

29 Ibid.

30 Ibid.

31 Purendra Prasad, "Introduction: Health Inequities in India – The Larger Dimensions", in *Equity and Access: Health Care Studies in India,* ed. Purendra Prasad and Amar Jessani (New Delhi: OUP, 2018).

32 "Financing and Delivery of Health Care Services in India," *National Commission on Macroeconomics and Health, Background Paper,* Ministry of Health & Family Welfare, Government of India (New Delhi: August 2005), 41.

33 Hooda, "Health System in Transition in India", 509–10.

34 See Imrana Qadeer, Kasturi Sen, and K.R. Nayar, ed. *Public Health and Poverty of Reforms* (New Delhi: Sage Publications, 2001).

35 "Delivery of Health Services in the Public Sector", *National Commission on Macroeconomics and Health, Background Paper,* Ministry of Health & Family Welfare, Government of India (New Delhi: August, 2005), 48. Also see David Peters, A. Yazbeck, R. Sharma, et al., "Better Health Systems for India's 'Financing and Delivery of Health Care Services in India'", *National Commission on Macroeconomics and Health, Background Paper*, Ministry of Health & Family Welfare, Government of

India (New Delhi: August, 2005); *Findings, Analysis and Options* (Washington, DC: World Bank, 2002); Charu C. Garg and Anup K. Karan, "Catastrophic and Poverty Impact of Out of Pocket Payment for Health Care in India: A State level Analysis", *Working Paper No. 23* (Institute for Human Development, 2004).

36   Rao, op. cit., 21.
37   Government of India, *Tenth Five Years Plan 2002–2007*, Vol. 2 (New Delhi: Planning Commission, 2002b).
38   Ibid.
39   *National Rural Health Mission, Meeting People's Health Needs in Rural Areas: Framework for Implementation 2005–2012* (New Delhi: Ministry of Health and Family Welfare, Government of India).
40   Ibid.
41   Government of India, *Prime Minister's Speech on Launch of NRHM* on 12 April 2005, accessed at http://www.pmindia.nic.in on 20.12.2021.
42   National Rural Health Mission, MoHFW, Government of India, 2005.
43   C. Lahariya, H. Khandekar, J. Prasuna, and Meenakshi, "A Critical Review of National Rural Health Mission in India", *The Internet Journal of Health* 6, no. 1 (2006): 1–4.
44   Ibid.
45   Ibid. For details of NRHM and ASHA see National Rural Health Mission, MoHFW, Government of India, 2005.
46   NRHM, MoHFW, Government of India, 2005.
47   Ibid. Also see NRHM, MoHFW, Government of India, 2005; Rao, *Do We Care?* 298–378; C. Lahariya, H Khandekar, J Prasuna, and Meenakshi, "A Critical Review of National Rural Health Mission in India", *The Internet Journal of Health* 6, no. 1 (2006): 1–4; A.K. Sharma, "The National Rural Health Mission: A Critique", *Sociological Bulletin* 63, no. 2 (May–August 2014): 287–301; Rajib Dasgupta and Imrana Qadeer, "The National Rural Health Mission (NRHM): A Critical Overview", *Indian Journal of Public Health* 49, no. 3 (2005): 138–40.
48   Imrana Qadeer, "Universal Health Care in India: Panacea for Whom?" http://www.ijph.in, accessed on 22.11.2021. Also see K. Srinath Reddy and Manu Raj Mathur, "Universal Health Coverage: How Viable?", in *Equity and Access: Health Care Studies in India*, ed. Purendra Prasad and Amar Jessani (New Delhi: OUP, 2018), 308–309.
49   Imrana Qadeer, "Universal Health Care: The Trojan Horse of Neoliberal Policies", *Social Change* 43, no. (June 2013): 149–64.
50   Vikas Bajpai and Anoop Saraya, "NRHM – The Panacea for Rural Health in India: A Critique", *Indian Journal of Public Health Research and Development* 1, no. 3 (2013): 24–30.
51   A. Wagstaff, M. Lindelow, G. Jun, X. Ling, and Q. Juncheng, "Extending Health Insurance to the Rural Population: An Impact Evaluation of China's New Cooperative Medical Scheme", *Journal of Health Economics* 28, no. 1 (2009): 1–19 and U. Giedion, E.A. Alfonso, and Y. Diaz, "The Impact of Universal Coverage Schemes in the Developing World: A Review of the Existing Evidence" (Universal Health Coverage (UNICO) Studies Series), Vol. 25 (Washington, DC: The World Bank, 2013) cited in Anup Karan, Winnie Yip, and Ajay Mahal, "Extending Health Insurance to the Poor in India: An Impact Evaluation of Rashtriya Swasthya Bima Yojana on Out of Pocket Spending for Healthcare" (nih.gov), *Social Science and Medicine* 181 (2017): 83–92, https://doi.org/10.1016/j.socscimed.2017.03.053, accessed on 28.11.2022. (Hereafter cited as Karan, Yip, amd Mahal, "Extending Health Insurance to the Poor in India").
52   Rajesh Kumar Sinha, "A Critical Assessment of Indian National Health Insurance Scheme – Rashtriya Swasthya Bima Yojana" (RSBY) 1, no. 8 (November 2013): 2305–306. (Hereafter cited as Sinha, "A Critical Assessment of Indian National Health Insurance Scheme").
53   Ibid.

54 https://main.mohfw.gov.in › files › 12Chapter, accessed on 28.11.2021.
55 Karan, Yip, and Mahal, "Extending Health Insurance to the Poor in India".
56 Sonalini Khetrapal and Arnab Acharya, "Expanding Healthcare Coverage: 'An Experience from RashtriyaSwasthyaBimaYojna'", – PubMed (nih.gov), accessed on 28.11.2021, Madhurima Nundy, Rajib Dasgupta, Kanica Kanungo, Sulakshana Nandi, and Ganapathy Murugan, "The Rashtriya Swasthya Bima Yojana (RSBY) Experience in Chhattisgarh: What Does it Mean for Health for All?", A paper published by SAMA: A Resource Group for Women and Health (New Delhi, 2013); R.A. Palacios, "New Approach to Providing Health Insurance to Poor in India: The Early Experience of Rashtriya Swasthya Bima Yojna", in *India's Health Insurance Scheme for the Poor: Evidence from the Early Experience of the Rashtriya Swasthya Bima Yojana,* ed. Palacious, Das, and Sun (New Delhi: Centre for Policy Research, 2011); S. Selvaraj and A. K. Karan, "Why Publicly-Financed Health Insurance Schemes are Ineffective in Providing Financial Risk Protection?" *Economic & Political Weekly* 47, no. 11 (2012): 460–68.
57 Karan, Yip, and Mahal, "Extending Health Insurance to the Poor in India".
58 A. Sinha, "Critical Assessment of Indian National Health Insurance Scheme", 2321.
59 Prasad, "Health Care Reforms", 57–59.
60 Ibid. Also see Rao, *Do We Care?*, 24–25.
61 https://www.niti.gov.in/planningcommission.gov.in/docs/sectors/health.php?sectors =health, accessed on 29.11.2021.
62 Ibid.
63 Ibid.
64 http://mohfw.nic.in/nrhm/Draft_Health_Bill/, accessed on 28.11.2021.
65 Ibid.
66 Ibid, also see accessed on 28.11.2021.
67 Imrana Qadeer and Indira Chakravarthi, "The Neo-Liberal Interpretation of Health", *Social Scientist* 38, no. 5/6 (May–June 2010): 50.
68 Imrana Qadeer, "Universal Health Care: The Trojan Horse of Neoliberal Policies", *Social Change* 43, no. 2 (2013): 154–55 (hereafter cited as Qadeer, "Universal Health Care: The Trojan Horse").
69 Ibid. For more details of National Health Bill, see "The Neo-Liberal Interpretation of Health", *Social Scientist* 38, no. 5/6 (May–June 2010).
70 Qadeer, "Universal Health Care: The Trojan Horse", 154.
71 Health Insurance in Andhra Pradesh was launched in 2007 by the state government covering about 70 million people (BPL households).
72 Rao, *Do We Care?*, 358.
73 A. Derickson, "Health Security for All? Social Unionism and Universal Health Insurance 1935–1958", *The Journal of American History* 80, no. 4 (1994): 1333–35, cited in K. Srinath Reddy and Manu Raj Mathur, "Universal Health Coverage: How Viable?" in *Equity and Access: Health Care Studies in India*, ed. Purendra Prasad and Amar Jessani (New Delhi: OUP, 2018), 305–306.
74 W. Beveridge, *Social Insurance and Allied Services* (London: H M Station Off, 1942), cited in K. Srinath Reddy and Manu Raj Mathur, "Universal Health Coverage: How Viable?", in *Equity and Access: Health Care Studies in India*, ed. Purendra Prasad and Amar Jessani (New Delhi: OUP, 2018), 305–306 (Hereafter cited as Reddy and Mathur, "Universal Health Coverage").
75 http://whqlibdoc.who.int/whr/2010/9789241564021_eng.pdf, accessed on 2.12.2021.
76 https://www.worldbank.org/en/topic/universalhealthcoverage#1, accessed on 2.12.2021.
77 For more details on PHFI see Rao, *Do We Care?*, 25.
78 Rao, op. cit., 58.
79 *High Level Expert Group Report on Universal Health Coverage for India*, Instituted by Planning Commission of India (New Delhi: November, 2011).

80   Ibid.
81   Reddy and Mathur," Universal Health Coverage", 312.
82   For details of the controversy regarding the HLEG report between the Planning Commission and Health Ministry see Rao, *Do We Care?*, 358–69.
83   *High Level Expert Group Report on Universal Health Coverage for India*, Instituted by the Planning Commission of India (New Delhi: November, 2011). Also see Imrana Qadeer, "Universal Health Care: The Trojan Horse of Neoliberal Policies", *Social Change* 43, no. (June 2013): 149–64.
84   Ravi Duggal, "A Financing Strategy for Universal Access to Health Care: Maharashtra Model", in *Equity and Access: Health Care Studies in India*, ed. Purendra Prasad and Amar Jessani (New Delhi: OUP, 2018), 312 (hereafter cited as Duggal, "A Financing Strategy for Universal Access to Health Care").
85   Planning Commission, *Social Sectors; Twelfth Five Year Plan (2012–2017)* (New Delhi: Planning Commission of India, 2013).
86   Reddy and Mathur, "Universal Health Coverage", 313.
87   Cited in Duggal, "A Financing Strategy for Universal Access to Health Care", 343–44.
88   Ibid., 345.
89   See Imrana Qadeer, "Universal Health Care: The Trojan Horse of Neoliberal Policies", 149–64. Also see Imrana Qadeer, "Universal Health Care in India: Panacea for Whom?" http://www.ijph.in, accessed on 22.11.2021. Also see Indranil Mukhopadhyay, "Universal Health Coverage: The New Face of Neoliberalism" *Social Change* 43 (2013): 177.
90   Rao, op. cit., 27.
91   Duggal, "A Financing Strategy for Universal Access to Health Care", 345.
92   Rao, op. cit., 366.
93   Ibid., 3–344, 367.
94   Ibid., 368.
95   Ibid., 369.
96   *National Health Policy 2015 Draft*, Ministry of Health & Family Welfare December, New Delhi (2014).
97   Government of India, *National Health Accounts 2004–05* (New Delhi: Ministry of Health and family Welfare, Government of India, 2009).
98   Reddy and Mathur, "Universal Health Coverage", 315.
99   NHP Draft 2015.
100 Ibid.
101 Reddy and Mathur, "Universal Health Coverage", 315–16.
102 Ibid.
103 Vikas Bajpai, "National Health Policy, 2017 Revealing Public Health Chicanery", *Economic and Political Weekly* LIII, no. 28 (July 2014): 31.
104 http://www.who.int/gho/publications/mdgs-sdgs/en/, World Health Organization, Health in 2015; From MDG's to SDGs. 2015, accessed on 1.12.2021.
105 For more details see, Situation Analyses, *Backdrop to the National Health Policy 2017*, Ministry of Health and Family Welfare, Government of India.
106 *National Health Policy 2017*, Ministry of Health and Family Welfare (New Delhi: Government of India).
107 Ibid.
108 Ibid.
109 Ibid.
110 Ibid.
111 Ibid.
112 Ibid.
113 Ibid.
114 Ibid.

115 Ibid.
116 For Critique of the NHP 2017 see Vikas Bajpai, "National Health Policy, 2017: Revealing Public Health Chicanery", *Economic and Political Weekly* LIII, no. 28 (July 2014); Rajiv Kumar Gupta and Rashmi Kumari, "National Health Policy 2017: An Overview", *Science* 19, no. 3 (July–September 2017); S. Sharma, et al., "National Health Policy 2017: Can It Lead to Achievement of Sustainable Development Goals?", https://www.researchgate.net/publication/322287585, accessed on 10.12.2021.
117 Nirupam Bajpai and Manisha Wadhwa, "Health and Wellness Centres: Expanding Access to Comprehensive Primary Health Care in India", *ICT India Working Paper #13*, Centre of Sustainable Development, Earth Institute, Columbia University (July 2019).
118 link.springer.com/article/10.1007/s12098-020-03359-z, accessed on 13.12.2021.
119 Website of National Health Authority, Government of India. For details of PM JAY see http://www.pib.gov.in/PressReleaseIframePage.aspx?PRID=1518544, accessed on 23.12.2021.
120 www.thehindu.com, accessed on 23.09.2018.
121 https://www.india.gov.in/, National Portal of India, Ayushman Bharat.

References

Bagchi, Amrita. "Reforms or Dictates: The Role of the Donor Agencies on Health Care in West Bengal". *Global South–Sephis e-Magazine* 7, no. 3. (July 2011): 34–45.

Bajpai, Nirupam, and Wadhwa Manisha. "Health and Wellness Centres: Expanding Access to Comprehensive Primary Health Care in India". *ICT India Working Paper #13*, Centre of Sustainable Development, Earth Institute, Columbia University (July 2019).

Bajpai, Vikas. "National Health Policy, 2017: Revealing Public Health Chicanery". *Economic and Political Weekly LIII*, no. 28 (July 2014): 31–35.

Baru, Rama V., and Madhurima Nundy. "Blurring of Boundaries: Public-Private Partnerships in Health Services in India". *Economic and Political Weekly* 43, no. 4 (January-February 2008): 114–125.

Dasgupta, Rajib, and Imrana Qadeer. "The National Rural Health Mission (NRHM): A Critical Overview". *Indian Journal of Public Health* 49, no. 3 (2005): 138–140.

Gangolli, Leena V., Duggal Ravi, and Shukla Abhay, eds. *Review of Healthcare in India*. Mumbai: Centre for Enquiry into Health and Allied Themes, 2005.

Garg, Charu C., and Anup K. Karan, "Catastrophic and Poverty Impact of Out of Pocket Payment for Health Care in India: A State Level Analysis". *Working Paper No. 23*. Institute for Human Development, 2004.

Government of India. *National Health Policy-2002*. New Delhi: Department of Health, Ministry of Health and Family Welfare, 2002a.

Government of India. *Tenth Five Years Plan 2002–2007*, Vol. 2. New Delhi: Planning Commission, 2002b.

Government of India. *National Rural Health Mission*. New Delhi: MoHFW, 2005.

Governemnt of India. *Prime Minister's Speech on Launch of NRHM*. 12 April 2005. Accessed at http://www.pmindia.nic.in.

Government of India. *National Health Accounts 2004–05*. New Delhi: Ministry of Health and family Welfare, 2009.

Government of India. *National Rural Health Mission, Meeting People's Health Needs in Rural Areas: Framework for Implementation 2005–2012*. New Delhi: Ministry of Health and Family Welfare, 2012.

Government of India. *Backdrop to the National Health Policy 2017*. New Delhi: Ministry of Health and Family Welfare, 2017.

Government of India. *National Health Policy 2017*. New Delhi: Ministry of Health and Family Welfare, 2017.

Gupta, Rajiv Kumar, and Rashmi Kumari. "National Health Policy 2017: An Overview". *JK Science* 19, no. 3 (2017).

High Level Expert Group Report on Universal Health Coverage for India. Instituted by Planning Commission of India. New Delhi: Planning Commission of India, November, 2011.

Hodges, Sarah, and Mohan Rao. *Public Health and Private Wealth: Stem Cells, Surrogates and Other Strategic Bodies*. Delhi: Oxford University Press, 2016.

Hooda, Shailendra. "Health System in Transition in India: Journey from State Provisioning to Privatization". *World Review of Political Economy* 11, no. 4 (Winter 2020): 506–532.

http://mohfw.nic.in/nrhm/Draft_Health_Bill.

http://www.who.int/gho/publications/mdgs-sdgs/en/, World Health Organization, Health in 2015; From MDG's to SDGs. 2015.

https://main.mohfw.gov.in › files › 12Chapter.

https://www.india.gov.in/, National Portal of India, Ayushman Bharat.

https://www.niti.gov.in/planningcommission.gov.in/docs/sectors/health.php?sectors =health.

Karan, Anup, Winnie Yip,and Ajay Mahal. "Extending Health Insurance to the Poor in India: An Impact Evaluation of Rashtriya Swasthya Bima Yojana on Out of Pocket Spending for Healthcare". *Social Science and Medicine* 181 (2017): 83–92.

Khetrapal, Sonalini, and Arnab Acharya. "Expanding Healthcare Coverage: An Experience from Rashtriya Swasthya Bima Yojna" *Indian Journal of Medical Research* 149, no. 3 (2019): 369–375.

Kurian, Oommen C., Suchitra Wagle, and Prashant Raymus. *Mapping the Flow of User Fees in a Public Hospital*. Bombay: Centre for Enquiry into Health and Allied Themes, 2011.

Lagardea, Mylene, and Natasha Palmer. "The Impact of User Fees on Health Service Utilization in Low- and Middle-Income Countries: How Strong is the Evidence." *Bulletin of the World Health Organization* 86, no. 11 April 2008: 839–848 (A–C).

Lahariya, C., H. Khandekar, J. Prasuna, and Meenakshi. "A Critical Review of National Rural Health Mission in India". *The Internet Journal of Health* 6, no. 1 (2006): 124.

link.springer.com/article/10.1007/s12098-020-03359-z.

Ministry of Health & Family Welfare. *National Health Policy 2015 Draft*. New Delhi: Ministry of Health & Family Welfare, 2014.

Ministry of Health & Family Welfare, Government of India. "Financing and Delivery of Health Care Services in India". *National Commission on Macroeconomics and Health*, Background Paper, New Delhi (August 2005).

Ministry of Health & Family Welfare. *National Health Policy 2015 Draft*. New Delhi: Ministry of Health & Family Welfare, 2014.

Mukhopadhyay, Alok. ed. *Report of the Independent Commission on Health in India*. New Delhi: Voluntary Health Associations of India, 1997.

Mukhopadhyay, Indranil. "Universal Health Coverage: The New Face of Neoliberalism". *Social Change* 43 (2013): 177–190.

Nandaraj, Sunil. "Beyond the Law and the Lord, Quality of Private Health Care". *Economic and Political Weekly* XXIX, no. 27 (1994): 1680–1685.

Nundy, Madhurima, Rajib Dasgupta, Kanica Kanungo, Sulakshana Nandi, and Ganapathy Murugan. *"The Rashtriya Swasthya Bima Yojana (RSBY) experience in Chhattisgarh: What does it mean for Health for All?"* A paper published by New Delhi: SAMA: A Resource Group for Women and Health, 2013.

Planning Commission, Government of India. *Eighth Five Year Plan Highlights.* New Delhi: Directorate of Advertising and Visual Publicity, Government of India, 1992.

Prasad, Purendra, and Amar Jesani, eds. *Equity and Access: Health Care Studies in India.* New Delhi: OUP, 2018.

Qadeer, Imrana. "Universal Health Care in India: Panacea for Whom?" http://www.ijph .in, 2013.

Qadeer, Imrana. "Universal Health Care: The Trojan Horse of Neoliberal Policies". *Social Change* 43 (June 2013): 149–164.

Qadeer, Imrana, and Indira Chakravarthi. "The Neo-Liberal Interpretation of Health". *Social Scientist* 38, no. 5/6 (May–June 2010): 49–51.

Qadeer, Imrana, Kasturi Sen, and K.R. Nayar, eds. *Public Health and Poverty of Reforms.* New Delhi: Sage Publications, 2001.

Rao, K. Sujatha. *Do We Care? India's Health System.* New Delhi: OUP, 2020.

Roy, Bijoya, and Siddharta Gupta. "Public-Private Partnership and User Fees in Healthcare: Evidence from West Bengal". *Economic and Political Weekly* xlvi, no. 38 (September 2011): 74–78.

Sharma, A.K. "The National Rural Health Mission: A Critique". *Sociological Bulletin* 63, no. 2 (May–August 2014): 287–301.

Sharma, S., A. Ghosh, and R. Pal. National Health Policy 2017: Can It Lead to Achievement of Sustainable Development Goals? https://www.researchgate.net/publication /322287585, 2018.

Sinha, Rajesh Kumar. "A Critical Assessment of Indian National Health Insurance Scheme – Rashtriya Swasthya Bima Yojana (RSBY)". *European Academic Research* 1, no. 8 (November 2013): 2299–2325.

Thomas, Sanjeev V. "The National Health Bill 2009 and Afterwards". Editorial, http:// www.annalsofian.org/ on Tuesday, May 1, 2018.

Website of National Health Authority, Government of India. For details of PM JAY. http:// www.pib.gov.in/PressReleaseIframePage.aspx?PRID=1518544.

West Bengal Health Policy Note. World Bank South Asia Region (June 2004).

World Bank. "India: Raising the Sights: Better Health Systems for India's Poor". *World Bank Report no. 22304.* Washington, DC: World Bank, 2001.

World Bank. *World Development Report 1993: Investing in Health.* New York: Oxford University Press,1993.

www.thehindu.com.

3 Public Health Sector and the Development of Nursing Homes in an Eastern Indian Metropolis

From Independence to Late 1990s

Introduction

Health status is integrally related to the socio-economic factors of a certain geographical space. It is needless to mention that the healthcare delivery services are also largely shaped by the socio-economic aspects. Rama V. Baru[1] has aptly pointed out that healthcare services are not mere technical interventions which exist in a vacuum, but are influenced by socio-economic issues.

From this perspective, we will focus on the development of public healthcare services (in Section I) and of nursing homes (in Section II) in the eastern Indian metropolis of Kolkata following the Independence of the country. Since the demographic shift is inextricably linked with the healthcare services, the pattern of population changes, especially the in-migration that Kolkata had experienced, posed a direct threat to healthcare delivery. Hence, the nature of healthcare, whether it is public or private, should be studied by taking into consideration all the adjoining factors, which will also throw some light on the existing healthcare culture of Kolkata.[2]

Section I

Situating Public Health and Healthcare Services in Kolkata – A General Outline

Though this study aims to discuss the private healthcare services of post-1947 Kolkata (earlier called Calcutta), a few words should be devoted to the public health condition of the city as well. An attempt should also be made to look into the public health and healthcare scenario of the Bengal (after Independence West Bengal) province, of which Kolkata is the capital city.

Conditions of Public Health in Colonial Period

The British seldom noted the ecological disturbances due to the expansion of communication through roads and railways, and at the same time neglected waterways such as canals and rivers, which for centuries had served the need of transportation. They often paid no heed to or did not realize the disastrous consequences to

DOI: 10.4324/9781003169475-4

the health of the people. By their careless operations, they created conditions for the progress of diseases and displacement. Communication networks also spread diseases; malaria is aptly called a disease of development.[3] Moreover, the building of railways started in the middle of the nineteenth century. The Calcutta-Ranaghat railroad was started in 1862 and by 1872 there were no less than 900 miles of railway tracks.[4] It is an interesting coincidence that every year the railways were built there were reports of fever epidemics in the Burdwan district. It was rightly said by K.C. Ghosh that the railways are a most prolific source of Anopheline breeding places and malaria of a virulent type.[5]

In a more recent study by Arabinda Samanta,[6] the deplorable conditions of public health and sanitation in colonial Bengal have been depicted. Closely connected with the phenomenon of deteriorating environment was the apathetic state of health and hygiene among the people in rural Bengal. This again stemmed from continued poverty and starvation over time. Increasing number of embankments and railways reduced the chances of flood and inundation. This in turn meant a progressive loss of fertility of the soil. Loss of soil fertility diminished the quantum of winter harvest, which meant starvation for the rural masses.[7]

Poor sanitation around the plantation areas created a micro-environment favourable for mosquito breeding and spreading malaria among the inhabitants. Thus, the expansion of irrigation canals, railroads and embankments created congenial habitat for malaria-carrying mosquitoes.[8]

Smallpox, locally known as *basanta rog*, was one of the major epidemic diseases in Bengal. Like most other infectious diseases, smallpox exhibited a seasonal incidence occurring mainly during the first half of the year. Calcutta seemed to serve as an important disseminating focus of smallpox infection where the epidemic of a serious nature once broke out in 1838 and again in 1848–1850 and 1856–1858. The disease acquired a deadly association with famine and prevailed in a severe epidemic form from 1943 to 1945.[9]

Actually, the outbreak of these diseases (malaria, cholera, smallpox, kala-azar, tuberculosis, leprosy) and infections were mainly the results of malnutrition and under-nutrition of the entire populace. Along with this, poor standards of nutrition, bad housing conditions and adulteration of foodstuff worsened the public health situation of Calcutta and contributed immensely to the ill health of the people. Calcutta was also deprived of the provision of safe drinking water. Kabita Ray has recorded that infant and maternal mortality was staggering.[10]

The real problem was however the apathy shown by the bureaucracy towards the problems of public health which were no doubt formidable, but not insoluble.[11] "The imperial government did not, of course, place sanitary reforms or medical services high on its list of priorities," admitted Roger Jeffrey.[12] What was essential was the formation of a dynamic outlook in regard to public health, the evils of which called for more thoroughgoing and varied efforts for their eradiation. But the public health policy of the government was characterized by vacillation.[13] Over the years, there has been a general tendency of neglect by the rulers of the country on health and healthcare issues. Both the colonial state and later the welfarist state have not taken the steps required to enable this sector to meet the needs of the country, which is densely populated and poverty-stricken.

Hospitals and Dispensaries in Bengal Presidency

The first hospital in Bengal was opened in early 1708 as indicated in the accounts of the *Early Annals of the English in Bengal*. It was mainly meant for the soldiers and seamen of the East India Company. Other Company servants could also avail themselves of its service. This hospital, within the Fort William precinct, was ruined during the battle between the Company and the Nawab of Bengal, Siraj-ud-Daulah, in 1757. The second hospital in Bengal Presidency was a temporary building erected inside the old Fort after the recovery of Calcutta by the Company. It was perhaps a makeshift hospital, carelessly managed with little space and free and open air. As a temporary measure, in October 1762, the Council agreed to build another hospital near Surman's gardens, i.e., Kidderpore. When the old fort was converted into a customhouse, it became absolutely necessary to build a new hospital. Therefore, a third hospital, which came to be known as the Presidency General Hospital, was built in 1769.

All these three hospitals were primarily intended for the Company's soldiers and sailors, but they also admitted Europeans of all classes and statuses. Presidency General Hospital was subsequently enlarged and surrounded by a wall, which afforded ample accommodation in separate buildings for patients and for the medical officers and establishments attached to the institution. This was in fact the first hospital where the construction, repair and maintenance cost was borne entirely by the colonial government. In 1792 the Company decided to open a hospital for the native poor in Bengal. Subsequently in 1792–1793 a hospital was erected in a house on the Chitpore Road. Both Europeans and Indians controlled it. The Presidency General Hospital was then exclusively meant for the Europeans. The native poor now flocked to the hospital meant for them. The popularity of the native hospital prompted the government to open another of its kind in 1794 at Dharmatola, which later became the Medical College Hospital in 1853.[14]

The *Journal of Indian Medical Association*, in a supplement published in 1948,[15] provided a short narrative on the hospitals in Calcutta. It describes the situation in the following manner.

A committee appointed by Lord William Bentinck in October 1833 recommended the establishment of the Calcutta Medical College on 1 February 1835 with the objective of 'supplying medical relief' to the general population and in particular to meet the demands of the various station hospitals. The Calcutta Medical College was supported by Ezra Hospital, the Prince of Wales Hospital, the Eden Hospital, the Eye Hospital, Sir J. Anderson Casualty Block, Chunilal Seal's Dispensary and Sisir Nibas. In addition there were special departments for skin, tuberculosis, ear, nose and throat, dental, venereal diseases, chest, X-ray and radium therapy. The total number of beds in the hospital was 809.[16]

In 1852, vernacular classes were introduced in the Medical College, which attracted a considerable number of students. In 1873, the vernacular class was transferred from Medical College to Sealdah which became the Campbell Medical School named after the then Lieutenant-Governor Sir George Campbell. So the school was the direct successor of the vernacular doctor class from the Medical College.[17]

The Justices of Peace for the town of Calcutta, the predecessors of the municipal commissioners, opened the Campbell Hospital, Sealdah, on 1 July 1867, as a popular hospital. On 1 December 1873, it was attached to the Campbell Medical School. This hospital was almost entirely rebuilt in 1908–1910. The hospital had 712 beds and provided a wealth of clinical materials for teaching purposes.[18]

A year later, in 1881, the Eden Hospital was opened. In 1882 it had 83 indoor patients of whom 42 were Indians and the rest were Europeans who were given better facilities. The emergencies of the 'Sepoy Mutiny' in 1857 compelled the Government to employ three female nurses at the Allahabad Military Hospital. The success of their performance led to the establishment of the Nurses' Training Institution in Calcutta for which the government sanctioned a capital grant of Rs 20,000 in 1876 for the construction of a building near the present Presidency General Hospital. Trained nurses were gradually employed in all the city hospitals. In the early twentieth century, the Calcutta Hospital Nurses' Institution undertook the recruitment, training and placement of the entire nursing staff in different hospitals in Calcutta. In 1897 the Sambhu Nath Pandit Hospital at Bhowanipur was opened. This hospital was built by contributions from the government, the Corporation of Calcutta and the funds of the old Sambhu Nath Pandit Outdoor Dispensary, which was absorbed into the new hospital. The Calcutta School of Tropical Medicine was founded in 1914 based on the lines of the London School of Tropical Medicine that had been established in London in 1899. The Europeans looked upon the tropics as a terrible place. The deaths and suffering of the White people from peculiar tropical diseases were matters of grave concern for the colonial authorities. In 1916 the Carmichael Hospital for Tropical Diseases was also established. The Lying-in Hospital, which was later absorbed into the Medical College Hospital, was constructed in 1840 with an outpatient dispensary and a training class for *dais* or native midwives. It was not until the beginning of the nineteenth century that hospitals for the general population were established in some of the mofussil (suburban) towns.[19]

The R.G. Kar Medical College, earlier known as Carmichael Medical College, was the first non-official recognized Medical College in India. It came into existence in 1916. The institution that developed into this college was at the time of affiliation known as the Calcutta Medical School and College of Physicians and Surgeons of Bengal. The college was named after Lord Carmichael in April 1919 and renamed R.G. Kar Medical College in 1947. Associated Hospitals of R.G. Kar Medical College were Albert Victor Hospital, Surgical Hospital, B.C. Dey Infectious Hospital, Nirmalendu Tuberculosis Hospital, Nalini Gupta Radium Annexe and Raja Debendra Nath Mullick Outdoor Dispensary. There were special departments for skin, tuberculosis, ear, nose and throat, dental, venereal diseases, mental diseases, cardiology, X-ray and radium therapy. The total number of beds in the hospital was 448.[20]

When the city was yet to have an infectious diseases hospital, there were wards in the Campbell Hospital for the treatment of smallpox, cholera and plague cases. Whenever an epidemic of these infectious diseases broke out, the Campbell Hospital was at the service of citizens and admitted hundreds of patients for necessary treatment. The Campbell Medical School and Hospital had the honour of being served by illustrious physicians like Sir U.N. Brahmachari, Sir Nilratan Sarkar, Sir Kedar Nath Das, Dr B.C. Roy and many others.[21]

The Lake Medical College with an attached 1,000-bed hospital in the Lake area was established on 1 April 1947 on a temporary basis by the Government of India. It was managed by the West Bengal government as the central government's agent for the training of ex-army medical licentiates undergoing a condensed M.B. course.[22]

Necessary arrangements for teaching anatomy, physiology and pharmacology were made in the Calcutta Medical College and R.G. Medical College. Clinical subjects and pathology were taught at the Lake Medical College.[23]

A fully equipped US Army Hospital situated in the Lake area was taken over for the purpose. The college and hospital were accommodated in the temporary buildings with cemented floors, single brick walls and tiled roofs and wards holding 30 beds were set up. There were gas and electric connections for a good kitchen, air-conditioned operation theatres and two air-conditioned wards. Sufficient equipment left by the Americans had been taken over for running the hospital.[24]

Arrangements were being made for the opening of self-contained anatomy, physiology and pharmacology departments within the Lake Medical College. Within a little over one year, the hospital had become very popular, but unfortunately it could not be extended due to a shortage of nursing staff.[25]

The Jatiya Ayurbijnan Parishad (National Medical Council) was founded in Calcutta in 1920 as a part of the national education movement. It started a teaching institution by the name of National Medical Institute on Wellington Street, which was later shifted to Maniktala Main Road where a large area of about 15 bighas of land was obtained from Maharaja Manindra Chandra Nandy of Cossimbazaar. A hospital was also established on the premises here and came to be known as the National Infirmary – a hospital for the poor and the destitute.[26]

Later, the organizers succeeded in obtaining a large area at its present site on Gorachand Road near Park Circus from the Calcutta Corporation on a nominal rent. A hospital with a three-storied building was built and it was named Chittaranjan Hospital. The National Infirmary was also maintained as a free hospital but the teaching section was transferred to Gorachand Road. Public support was not lacking at the time and very soon the association secured further area and built the present spacious two-storied building for the institute. A large dissection hall along with necessary auxiliary accommodation was also built. The buildings were constructed with a view to cater to the requirements of a medical college. No aid from the government at the time was available either for the school or for the hospital and the teachers; physicians and surgeons gave voluntary service.[27]

The Calcutta Medical Institute was established in 1922. Dr S.K. Mallik and his associates started a medical institution called National Medical College of India with a hospital then called King's Hospital at its present site on Upper Circular Road. The association of Calcutta Medical Institute with Jatiya Ayurbijnan Parishad actually had the objective of establishing another medical college which would commence its journey from 1948.[28]

Apart from the development of hospitals in the Bengal Presidency, there was also a large body of dispensaries serving the ailing population. Medical historians[29] of South Asia have paid little or no attention to the growth of this sector. Christian Hochmuth has rightly suggested that the Bengal dispensaries provided a unique glimpse into the colonial public health establishment due to the significant role it afforded to 'indigenous practitioners'. In other words, analyzing dispensary practice in South Asia allows us an unprecedented insight into the interaction between western and indigenous medicine.[30]

The establishment of charitable dispensaries from the 1830s was one of the earliest attempts to provide western medical care for the Indian people. Dispensaries became local centres for vaccination against smallpox and for conveying western ideas about sanitation and hygiene, and agencies for 'local sanitary amendments such as the digging of tanks and wells, fencing them off, and filling up holes'. This led to the opening of dispensaries in different parts of Bengal as well as in Calcutta. Many of these dispensaries owed their existence to Indian philanthropists, who provided the money for the building of dispensary houses and also a monthly sum for their maintenance. By the 1860s, the contribution from these philanthropists started declining. Hence, in some cases, the government provided them with 'native doctors' and medicines. Sometimes they were helped by commercial organizations like the Bengal Coal Company or by subscriptions from Europeans. However, from 1870, as an attempt to reduce public expenditure, the colonial administration sought to distance itself from the running of dispensaries, which it felt should rely increasingly on local funds. However, the total number of such institutions increased considerably in the decades after 1870.

Though the foundations of public hospitals were set up in colonial Calcutta, the quality of services they provided with their limited infrastructure was unsatisfactory.

"Some two decades ago, there were people who considered going to hospital as going away for good. Meanwhile, the number of hospitals has increased; there are more doctors, nurse-sisters, scientific equipment and medicine producing companies in the country and Calcutta. Still, the human factor in this unique institution of organized charity has little changed. Even today sisters are less sisterly healers are more like dealers and patients more impatient."

"A recent probe into some of the Principal Calcutta hospitals reveals the terrific amount of overcrowding and the consequent strain that are eating into the very basis that sustains a hospital spirit – the spiritual factor of human element. Equipments and accommodation remaining nearly constant, hospitals are today as much over crowded as are tramcars and dwelling houses in their own spheres."[31]

"Patients are accommodated by placing cots anywhere and everywhere, in the corridor, back spaces and in between already crowded rows; cases sprawl on the floor; there are many who have to be refused admission, however deserving the cases may be. Sometimes, blanket supplies go short and stricken people shiver when it is cold."

Absence of Human Relationship[32]

"The absence of humanness – sympathy – which is what is meant by hospital spirit. Besides, the average rough behaviour, harsh words and delaying officialdom on the part of hospital personnel (including menials) are too common in public knowledge to merit repetition.

Empty words have never bettered efficiency. When the society does not recognise in material terms the dignity and value of a service, the same non-recognition returns to the society like a boomerang, and as such one is paid in the same coins.

Ask any hospital administrator and he would reply: We want money to provide for more hospital personnel, more accommodation, medicines, diet and apparatus and comfort. But who is to foot the bill?

One of the administrators with 15 years experience in hospitals said: 'Hospital accommodation in Calcutta must be increased by at least five times the present one. If the Government cannot nationalize all of them, it must be seen that national funds are well distributed. The days of laissez-faire are gone.

The state can no longer shirk its responsibility and it is time it intervened. We take below the cases of some of the worst affected hospitals in Calcutta."

R.G. Kar Medical Hospital[33]

"Formerly known as Carmichael Medical College after the name of the then Governor Lord Carmichael, this 61-year-old hospital is one of the oldest medical hospitals. Beginning with a very modest number of 14 beds, it has now 531 beds, spread over surgical, medical, gynaecological, maternity, cholera, tuberculosis, ophthalmic, ENT and infectious disease wards. The number of beds has been stationary since 1944.

Every year, the number of patients treated increases by several thousands till it now comes to about one lakh, outdoors and indoors together. The number of students has increased from 60 in 1916 to more than 1,000 this year. Simultaneously has increased, as it would be, the annual expenditure now running to about 4½ lakhs of Rupees.

But it is curious to observe that the government grant to this hospital has remained the same (Rs 50,000) since 1918. However in 1918 West Bengal Premier Dr B. C. Roy has of course promised some financial help on the condition that the hospital demands nothing next five years.

The consequences of a hospital running a deficit of Rs 1,70,000 (last year) can easily be imagined.

Bed sheets are not regularly washed and some are as ancient as half a century. While on round in one of the indoor medical wards, flies were seen collecting on dirty beds with a sickening stink coming from somewhere somehow. There is no sufficient disinfectant available to the management. Some of the patients were found resting heads on what can be said to be an apology for pillows.

Similarly, the lack of funds has told upon the quantity and quality of diet, and medicines and services made available to patients.

Most often, patients themselves had to buy their own medicines, that too generally three times the actual needs. Moreover, medicines have a peculiar way of being spirited away from the cupboards. And those who cannot pay for them have to be content with sodi-bicarb mixtures.

A male nurse said:

What we do to patients is, let me say, nothing. Take, for instance, the business of washing patients' heads. You are given only one coolie and one *methar* and there are so many heads to wash. But who is to draw so much water? You cannot blame me if I have to satisfy myself with one jug of water for, say, three heads.

That is how a patient suffers from a shortage of manpower.

Students want better hostels, library, common rooms and playgrounds. They must have more and modern apparatus so that they can learn the modern way of treatment.

One can hardly believe when students complain that for blood examination, 100 students have only one hemocytometer to share. In the clinical laboratory, they have only four microscopes in all.

Take the eye testing outdoors for 80 patients a day, the department has only one set of refraction glasses.

Shortage in nursing hands compels a nurse to 'take care' of 30 patients at a time, doing duty for over 10 hours a day. He or she has not, so-to-say, a day off to relax. The number of permanent nursing staff is too little to cope with the hospital's demands."

Poor Scale of Pay[34]

"The poor scales of pay that the authorities have for their employees will be evident from the following:

Jokhan Jamadar of the Lower Subordinate Staff, now putting 25 years' service, earns <u>Rs 20/8/-</u> a month. Female sweepers, Janaki and Susila—with 35 years' service to credit—are each paid Rs 18/8/- a month. Head Compounder A. Ghosh's salary has risen from Rs 50 to 100 in 35 years while his subordinate compounders earn Rs 68 monthly, service period varying from 20 to 22 years.

The picture is similar in cases of mechanics, carpenters, tailors, liftmen, darwans, clerks and others.

A spokesman of the employees said they had demanded adequate wage increase, security of service, proper leave rules, accommodation and allowances, promotion rules, special requirements for nurses and lower-subordinate staff, proper working hours etc.

But it is always the vicious circle started by the overall lack of funds. If there is no money, what can the hospital administration do to meet the demands?

If neither the government, nor public bodies, nor the rich would agree to part with a portion of their sparable income, who will stand in the way of handing the patients over to the wolves?

The Development Committee has chalked out a development plan of its own, its present needs are estimated at about Rs 34,00,000, with a call for Rs 30,00.000 as reserve fund."

In the words of the Administration 'The authorities now face the tremendous difficulty to arrange proper diet and essential medicines for the patients'.

Campbell Medical Hospital[35]

"Though now a government hospital, the story is not much otherwise here too. While on the one hand there is universal demand for more doctors, nurses and menials, the existing personnel smarting under heavy overcrowding of patients, complain of hard work and underpay.

The nature of overcrowding can be seen from figures in the following excerpts:

The Surgical and Gynaecological Wards have 314 beds. The extras here come to about 148, a daily average, while the Medical Ward runs averagely 102 extras, beds numbering 158. It, therefore, did not appear strange when cots were laid on both sides of the Surgical Ward's verandah to accommodate the patients."

The most ill-reputed is perhaps the Infectious Ward from where none is refused admission. But the condition here is anything but inspiring. Some time ago, a senior staff nurse of the Kolkata Corporation was reported to have remarked, after an official had asked her why she did not remove herself to Campbell (she had an attack of cholera) "Do you think I should go to the Campbell knowing very well what the conditions are there?". With epidemics a permanent guest in the city, nothing short of an Infectious Diseases Hospital can withstand the needs of the populace.

"Only one Staff Nurse is sometimes entrusted with the charge of the whole of a ward, if not more. Dearth of nursing hands has made sisters to evolve a short-cut to all duty items they perhaps regard themselves as just wage-earners."

Chittaranjan Seva Sadan[36]

"The hospital is exclusively for women and children. The hospital was created to perpetuate the memory of Deshabandhu C. R. Das and has been presently carrying on with a pressure of 150 per cent over its actual accommodation. The number of outpatients treated last year is estimated to have neared about 50,000 while that of indoor admissions was about 7,000.

The hospital is going to have a cancer department of its own, which when completed, will be the only of its kind in the whole of Asia including Australia. The hospital needs about 30 lakhs of rupees for this, of which about eight lakhs have now been raised from public donations. The department expects a more generous response from the public."

The Lake Hospital[37]

"As the youngest of Kolkata hospitals, this is believed to be one of the best-equipped hospitals in India. The entire burden is borne by the Governments of India and West Bengal with an annual grant of 28 lakhs of rupees. Of this, the whole expenditure of the college side (Rs 5 lakhs) and 50 per cent of the hospital side (Rs 23 lakhs) is shouldered by the Centre.

The Government of West Bengal will decide after five years' time if the hospital will be run entirely by the West Bengal government on a permanent basis.

It has 583 beds and is presently running 49 extras. The average number of outdoor patients in different sections is about 900 a day and the diet supplied to patients is worth Rs 2 per capita per day."

Saying that the hospital is working under pressure in the medical and gynaecological sections, an official complained of the slowness of the government's engineering department in carrying out necessary construction repairs, saying that 'the red-tapism today is the same as it was during the British Raj'.

This narrative on the public hospitals of Kolkata throws some light on the issue that the degeneration of the services in government hospitals is not a recent development.

The state of healthcare was in a sorry state from the time of its inception. It was inadequate, ill-equipped and inefficient in both colonial and post-Independence times. An overview of the system reveals that despite its professed commitment to serve all – especially the poor – it was riddled with unevenness and inequalities.[38] In spite of the quantitative growth of the healthcare infrastructure, the medical services were made available to a tiny selected segment of the urban population. Qualitatively and quantitatively, public healthcare was poor and inadequate compared to the demand in Calcutta.

Public Health in Calcutta after Independence

Independence of India did not bring about any encouraging change in the public health scenario and the situation further worsened with the lack of improvement in hygiene and sanitary conditions. Public health, Amartya Sen and Jean Dreze argue, has been, 'One of the most neglected aspects of development in India'.[39] The poor pattern of investment in public health has resulted in a deplorable condition of the entire health and healthcare infrastructure.

After 1947, it has been observed that except for some progress during the First Five Year Plan in controlling malaria and improving the health services to some extent and in some provinces, the public health conditions in India were none too encouraging.[40]

In the XIII Bengal Provincial Medical Conference held in Midnapore, Dr A.K. Bose as the president of the conference referred to the prevailing health situation in India:

> But the position today is far from satisfactory and the result is that in India every year about 10 lakhs of people die of malaria, 5 lakhs of tuberculosis, 2 lakhs of dysentery, 1 lakh of cholera, 1 lakh of small pox and many lakhs of other diseases directly or indirectly related to malnutrition. Infant mortality is colossal; almost 50% of average mortality amongst children below the age of ten. A large percentage of those that somehow grow up become a source of economic drainage to the nation due to perpetual ill health.[41]

The diseases which were predominant in these decades had their origin in the British period. Since the conditions of hygiene and sanitation were far from satisfactory, the waterborne and communicable diseases such as malaria, filariasis, cholera, diarrhoeal diseases, leprosy, tuberculosis, etc. spread like an epidemic.

The First World War, the Bengal Famine and the Second World War disrupted the stability of the metropolis whose civic facilities were taxed beyond endurance.[42] All uncommitted vacant land in and around the city became the encampments of millions of homeless men and women. Thus hundreds of 'refugee colonies' sprang up almost overnight all around the city and occupied all the vacant land in the fringe areas. Here the refugees built their own type of settlement, bearing some reflection of the village set-up of their lost home. Thus, before the Calcutta Improvement Trust (CIT) could cross its own administrative hurdle – confinement to the municipal limits of the city – the refugees had taken command of the adjoining areas and transformed them into a very different environment. These settlements posed a massive challenge to the planning and development of the city in the following decades.[43]

By the 1950s, Calcutta's civic facilities were under severe strain and grossly inadequate. At the same time, Calcutta was beset by cholera epidemics, which drew the attention of the World Health Organization. In 1959, WHO deputed a consultant team led by Dr Abel Wolman to examine the water supply and environmental sanitation of Calcutta. The team highlighted the urgent need for rehabilitation and improvement of the water supply and environmental sanitation system. As the team also pointed out, the region of endemic cholera in India fell mainly within the state of West Bengal, with its nucleus in Greater Calcutta, and the cholera situation there had great significance not only for India but for the world at large.[44]

Along with this, mention should be made about the health status of the 'inheritors of slum and pavement life in Kolkata'.[45] This one-third of the city's population had multiplied more abundantly than they died. They worked for the benefit of the upper classes of Kolkata and undertook the most taxing occupations. They were sickly, malnourished and sometimes utterly destitute. Most of them had adopted a half-urban lifestyle illustrating a special history and social mobility.[46]

Unfortunately, these 24 lakh slum dwellers of Kolkata nominally benefited from the efforts of the CMDA. They lined out their monsoons among lanes in knee-deep mud, thick with garbage, chemicals and gobbets of flesh and hide. Inevitably with each monsoon, the area became a seedbed for enteric fever and malaria and some sporadic cases of malaria.[47]

Although urbanization is one of the indicators of development, very fast urbanization in developing countries has created problems of the proliferation of slums.

As a metropolis in a newly independent country, Calcutta had witnessed rapid changes in the demographic pattern. Moreover, the greater part of the migrants were poor and resourceless people who gathered in slums and shanty towns and even on roads and open spaces, creating new vicious environmental cycles of which they themselves were the chief victims. Acute urban poverty is reflected in its Physical Quality of Life Index (PQLI), which takes note of longevity, child mortality, shelter, availability of water, sanitation, educational facilities, power supply and health.[48]

Health hazards affected the well-being of not only the slum dwellers but also the affluent sections of the society in a different manner. Over the years, the predominance of lifestyle diseases or non-communicable diseases threatened the life of people living in the upper economic strata.[49]

Whatever steps had been taken, either in towns or in the rural areas, were not only grossly insufficient but equally unsatisfactory. The population of West Bengal was 2,4810,308 according to the 1951 census. The number of hospital beds was about 18,000. It roughly worked out to seven beds per 1,000 of the population, as compared to 11 and eight beds respectively in the USA and UK. Dr Trivedi pointed out that it was a disproportionate situation since the sickness incidence in India was definitely much higher than those of the other countries mentioned.[50]

Similarly, in the presidential address to the 13th Bengal Provincial Medical Conference held at Midnapore on 7 and 8 November 1953, Dr A.K. Basu said that West Bengal had about 16,000 qualified medical personnel. Of them, 7,000 were in the rural areas and about 9,000 were in the urban areas. So, in the rural areas, there were roughly about one doctor for 2,800 people, which made it difficult for rendering efficient medical relief even if proper institutional facilities were made available. Though in the urban areas the proportion was satisfactory, the doctors were being forced to leave not only the state but even the country in search of a better income. Even highly qualified specialists were doing the same. Basu remarked that on the one hand there was a shortage of doctors and on the other, they were being compelled to leave the state as there were not enough suitable places to employ them.[51]

Dr B.P. Trivedi, in his presidential address to the XVII Bengal Provincial Medical Conference at Bishnupur in 1958, observed that owing to various socio-economic factors and more consciousness, people were flocking to the hospitals. Naturally, the load was tremendous and the entire machinery had gone to pieces. The enquiry was no more for any bed but for a space. The sick and the suffering people were simply crowded together in beds on the floor making it impossible even for the doctors, nurses and others to move in the wards. Such a state of affairs had brought in another complication, namely defective teaching. Intimately connected with the overcrowding of the city hospitals was the condition of the district, sub-divisional and *thana* hospitals. For some years, the health department of the West Bengal government had been contemplating to upgrade the district and other hospitals with various specialities, but it was strange that the government had taken about ten years to decide whether such a scheme should be put into effect.[52]

Some administrators and planners had declared from time to time that they did not have the adequate number of doctors to man the hospitals, clinics and health centres and that therefore, the state must re-introduce a lower cadre of medical training, which the whole medical profession in India unanimously opposed. This should be examined in the context of West Bengal which possessed the largest number of health centres.[53]

The Bengali daily *Anandabazar Patrika* dated 30 October 1967[54] reported that there had been rapid spread of malaria in the adjoining areas of Calcutta. Blood tests, in almost 70 per cent cases, revealed the presence of the malarial parasite. What is important for our study is that this particular news report also recorded that people residing in these areas had never experienced the outbreak of malaria even ten years back. The degeneration of the entire hygiene and sanitary conditions undoubtedly resulted in the outbreak of this communicable disease.

Another interesting report published in *Anandabazar Patrika* on 12 November 1967[55] stated 'Malaria has emerged once again from the oblivion'. Measures were taken by the state health department to resist the rapid spread of the disease.

A brief report published in *Anandabazar Patrika* on 3 May 1967[56] stated that there had been rapid spread of cholera in the city. Hospitals all over the metropolis started admitting patients affected by cholera. More than 39 patients had been diagnosed with cholera and admitted in different city hospitals.

Various issues of the *Health on the March*[57] published during this period reported the deaths mostly from diseases such as cholera, smallpox, malaria, pulmonary tuberculosis and dysentery. In the 1971 issue of the *Health on the March*,[58] a report came of a new disease – diphtheria – that had broken out in the city. Maternal death and infant mortality were also predominant.[59]

Health Care in Calcutta after Independence

The first issue of *Health on the March*[60] provided data on the state of West Bengal as a whole. According to this, there were three categories of hospitals in urban areas (see Table 3.1):

Table 3.1 Distribution of Medical Institutions and Beds

Year	State		State-Aided		State Special	
	Number	Beds	Number	Beds	Number	Beds
1948	219	10,837	22	2,635	52	2,279
1949	232	11,533	22	2,856	50	2,233
1950	274	10,997	22	3,099	52	2,241
1951	288	10,057	22	3,099	52	2,247
1952	310	10,268	25	3,929	53	2,411
1953	335	10,975	27	3,879	59	2,411
1954	344	12,022	28	3,998	59	2,409
1955	380	12,991	33	4,779	60	2,409
1956	419	13,848	32	4,802	60	2,409
1957	446	14,170	31	5,212	59	2,407

Source: *Health on the March* (1948-1957), West Bengal (corrected up to 31 December 1957): Progress of Medical Institutions (hospitals only).

(i) State
(ii) State-aided
(iii) State special

In 1957, *Health on the March* recorded that West Bengal had a population of 28,488,196 with an area of 34,205 sq. miles. Apart from the hospitals which are listed above, there were also health centres, dispensaries and clinics in the rural belt of the various districts of West Bengal.

Despite all these efforts to build the health infrastructure, the healthcare conditions in Calcutta presented a picture of failure and steep decline in services, culminating in the present state of its serious sickness. Even in the 1950s, a senior physician had described the existing set-up as 'absolutely out of date for the present needs'.[61]

The 1962 issue of the *Health on the March* provided for the first time district-wise data of medical institutions. This data provide a detailed picture of the number and categories of hospitals and hospital beds.

The total number of hospitals, dispensaries and clinics and beds by districts in West Bengal as on 31st December 1962 are as follows (see Table 3.2):[62]

Though there are certain ambiguities in this classification (due to the confusion of the health department regarding this classification and subsequent clarification of each categories), this categorization continued with some alterations in the following period. In 1963, the category of 'private aided' had been replaced by 'state-aided' and there had been a reduction only in the total number of hospital beds. However, till 1972,[63] a similar classification continued with a subsequent increase in the number of hospitals and hospital beds (see Tables 3.3 and 3.4).

The tables explain that from 1962 to 1972, there had been a marginal increase in the number of hospitals below which was only 5.26 per cent. The number of

Table 3.2 Total Number of Hospitals and Beds in Calcutta as on 31 December 1962

	State		A.G & F.R.E.[a]		Local Fund		Private Aided		Private Non-Aided		Railway		State Special		Total	
	Number	Beds	Number	Beds	Number	Beds	Number	Beds	Number	Beds	Number	Beds	Number	Beds	Number	Beds
	11	5,045	1	200	7	308	23	3,146	6	290	3	180	5	556	57	9,745

A.G & F.R.E., Auxiliary Government and Famine Relief Emergency Hospitals.

Table 3.3 Public Healthcare Establishments in Calcutta

State		A.G & F.R.E.*		Local Fund		State-Aided		Private Non-Aided		State Special		Railways		Total	
Number	Beds	Number	Beds	Number	Beds	Number	Beds	Number	Beds	Number	Beds	Number	Beds	Number	Beds
17	7,355	1	100	8	391	17	2,586	10	476	5	638	2	335	60	11,901

Twenty-five years after Independence, the question of population increase and the expansion of healthcare infrastructure did exhibit an encouraging scenario in the context of the Calcutta Municipal Corporation area only.

Table 3.4 Estimated Mid-Year Population
by Districts (Calcutta)

Year	Population
1960	29,44,583
1961	29,06,342
1962	29,27,371
1963	29,80,125
1964	30,03,556
1965	30,26,436
1966	30,49,316
1967	30,72,196
1968	30,95,076
1969	31,17,956
1970	31,41,180

Source: *Health on the March* (various years).

Table 3.5 Year-wise Increase in Hospitals and Hospital Beds in Calcutta

Year	Increase in the Total No. of Hospitals	Increase in the Total No. of Hospital Beds
1962	57	9,745
1963	55	9,758
1964	54	10,467
1965	56	10,546
1966	58	10,938
1967	62	12,023
1968	62	12,002
1969	62	12,002
1970	62	12,182
1971	61	11,716
1972	60	11,901

hospital beds on the other hand had registered a growth of 22.12 per cent between 1962 and 1972. The estimated mid-year population of Calcutta (Table 3.5) from 1960 to 1970 expanded up to 7 per cent. On that basis, the population served per bed in the Calcutta Municipal Corporation (CMC) area was 258:1. This ratio was not much depressing in the 1960s and 1970s as far as the infrastructure of public healthcare is concerned.

But, the CMC area was closely surrounded by the Calcutta Urban Agglomeration (CUA) and Calcutta Metropolitan District (CMD).[64] The population of these two areas were 9.2 million and 10.1 million respectively and the economic activities in these areas were inseparable from the CMC area. Hence, the healthcare sector of the CMC area was also responsible for serving the population of the outer areas. The huge dependence threatened not only the healthcare services of the inner city but also exposed the inadequacy of the infrastructure. Interestingly, most of the patients in the public hospitals came from a rural or semi-urban background. Since public hospitals were the only resort in critical cases, even the affluent sections of the society utilized their services. The faith in the services of government hospitals and the doctors working there was still deep-rooted. The doctor–patient relationship was not influenced by commercial transactions.

Anandabazar Patrika of 22 May 1967[65] reported that the government was taking initiatives to nationalize Calcutta National Medical College and Chittaranjan Hospital. The then state health minister Nani Bhattacharya had expressed his willingness in the Cabinet and the decision would be soon accepted by the government. In the inauguration ceremony of Baranagar Hospital, Bhattacharya had declared that the government for their efficient functioning would take over the health centres that developed under private initiatives. Initially, the government had decided to take over National Medical College and Chittaranjan Seva Sadan for ten years. It was estimated that the state government would have to invest Rs 50 lakh in a year for nationalizing these two hospitals.

In June 1967, the state government finally issued an ordinance nationalizing National Medical College and Chittaranjan Hospital,[66] initially for ten years. Dr N.K. Biswas was made the administrator of both the college and the hospital.[67]

Among other state hospitals, special mention may be made of the Beliaghata Infectious Diseases Hospital which was started during the First Five Year Plan and completed during the Second Plan at a total cost of Rs 65.42 lakhs. It was one of the most up-to-date hospitals for the treatment of infection cases in India. The hospital had 280 permanent beds and there was provision for the accommodation of 540 temporary beds during the epidemic seasons. Within the same premises, a general hospital had also been started with 320 beds.[68]

In an autobiography by the veteran physician Dr Mani Kumar Chhetri, a narrative of the development of healthcare infrastructure in post-Independence Kolkata is wonderfully depicted. Dr Chhetri has brought out the fact that after Independence, health received proper attention from the welfare state and during Dr Bidhan Roy's regime, West Bengal witnessed multiple and far-reaching changes in the sphere of healthcare. With the assistance of AIIMS, modern dialysis units were introduced in different medical colleges in Calcutta. Indeed, the Coronary Care Unit (CCU) in SSKM for serious heart patients was set up in 1965 to reduce mortality rates caused by cardiac problems. Dr Chhetri has recalled that a few years later it was felt that patients suffering from any fatal disease should be placed in the Intensive Treatment Unit (ITU) which was renamed Critical Care Unit (CCU). The establishment of the trauma care unit for road accident cases was also an important achievement in the healthcare sector. In this way, modernized techno-centric approaches to health care were welcomed.[69]

In addition to the expansion of the existing state hospitals and the construction of new ones, the government also took over many important private hospitals. Some of these were:

(i)   The Lady Dufferin Victoria Hospital
(ii) The R.G. Kar Medical College and Hospital

(iii) The Sagar Dutta Hospital, Kamarhati

(iv) The B.C. Roy Polio Clinic and Hospital for crippled children, Beliaghata[70]

Government and non-government hospitals existing at that time in Calcutta were:[71]

   (i) Medical College Hospital

  (ii) NRS Medical College Hospital

 (iii) SSKM Hospital

 (iv) S.N. Pandit Hospital

  (v) Lady Dufferin Victoria Hospital

 (vi) R.G. Kar Hospital

(vii) M.R. Bangur Hospital

Non-government organizations working in the health sector were:

    (i) Ramakrishna Mission Seva Pratisthan

   (ii) Islamia Hospital

  (iii) Chittaranjan Hospital

  (iv) Balananda Brahmachari Hospital (Behala)

   (v) K.S. Roy T.B. Hospital (Jadavpur)

  (vi) Four Calcutta Corporation chest clinics

 (vii) Niramoy (Bhowanipore)

(viii) Niramoy (Ganesh Chandra Avenue)

  (ix) T.B. Relief Association (Dharmatolla Street)

   (x) Servants of Humanity Society (Upper Chitpur Road)

  (xi) Social Welfare Organisation

 (xii) Marwari Relief Society

(xiii) Garden Reach Chest Clinic

(xiv) Mayor's Chest Clinic

 (xv) Students' Health Home

(xvi) Paschim Banga Samaj Seba Samity

Swasthya Dwipika,[72] a Bengali journal on health and medical care, in an article titled *Sahar Kolkatar Katha* (story of the city of Kolkata) illustrated the healthcare conditions of the metropolis. This article provided the names of some other government and private hospitals and mentioned that the city had 15 hospitals with 500 indoor beds. Two of the private organizations were the Institute of Child Health at Dilkhusha Street and Lohia Matri Sadan. There were other hospitals like B.R. Singh Railway Hospital, Port Commissioner's Hospital and Lumbini Park Mental Hospital, which was the only private hospital treating mental patients in Calcutta. The Chittaranjan Cancer Hospital was established during this period. Afternoon pay clinics were opened in three of the governmental hospitals. A diagnostic clinic and a polyclinic were set up at the residence of Dr Bidhan Chandra Roy. A hospital was established in Narkeldanga in memory of

Dr Roy.[73] Another polyclinic affiliated with the Presidency General Hospital was opened at Bhowanipore. There were also numerous small clinics scattered all over the city.

Though the public healthcare facilities in Kolkata have exhibited a growth pattern in terms of bed strength and institutions, it was still inadequate to serve the needs of the population. In 1975, there were 61 healthcare institutions in the public sector and the number of beds was 12,873. In 1983, the number of hospitals and the bed strength increased to 66 and 15,260, respectively. The hospitals in the public sector increased to 77 and the number of beds to 18,899 in 1999.[74]

> Often no hospital or clinic is to be found within miles in rural areas. Even safe drinking water for the village people is still a dream after seven decades of Independence. The rural areas cannot hope to have even one doctor for every 20,000 population. It is therefore not at all difficult to understand how many people of our country are beyond the scope of the so-called existing healthcare system. Again, for those who have health centres and hospitals within their reach, there prevails a reign of 'NO' – no supply of oxygen, no bed vacant, no scope of urgent investigation. There is always a dearth of doctors, sisters and other staff. The number of sanctioned posts is far short of the requirement as per population, and yet kept largely vacant. Thus the doctors and nurses are perplexed with the rush of the patients.[75] There are thousands of doctors and other health workers unemployed and unutilized while diseased, millions are dying for lack of proper treatment.[76]

The following excerpts would illustrate the state of nursing services, a vital component of health services, in the city:

> At the Calcutta Medical College and Hospital the number of sanctioned beds is 2150 and the total strength of nursing staff is 459. The nurse-patient ratio thus comes around 1:5 as prescribed ideal by West Bengal Government (Government of West Bengal, Department of Health 1957).[77] But this is not the reality. Patients are admitted not according to beds. Very often more than one patient is accommodated in a single bed; even in the maternity ward, the prospective mothers with infant babies have to share a bed. One of the nurses of Calcutta Medical College and Hospital said that 'she alone was looking after 105 women admitted to the two wards'. Moreover, a good number of patients lie on the floor for the lack of hospital beds. In the emergency wards also, patients remain on the floor. So the actual number of patients admitted far exceeds the number of sanctioned beds. This apart from the entire nursing staff is not composed of only staff nurses, who have the normal duty of taking care of patients. Sister tutors are engaged in teaching. Nursing superintendents, Deputy nursing superintendents are in the administration. Matrons supervise the staff nurses who are directly related to indoor patients. In all twenty one nurses are engaged in teaching and administration. Again there are nurses who are in outdoor duty, X-ray units, operation theatres.[78]

Ten percent of the total nurses are on long leave (maternity or medical leave) throughout the year. So the exact number of working nurses came down to 393. Nursing service is again divided into three shifts. So the actual number of nurses working in the wards at any time is 393/3 = 131. Where the actual number of patients is around 2,500, the nurse–patient ratio is 131:2,500 = 1:19. Even if the number of patients does not exceed the number of sanctioned beds, then also the nurse–patient ratio comes under 1:17, the standard during 1987 set for nurse–patient ratio was 1:3. So the nurses of Calcutta Medical College and Hospital are working against an adverse nurse:patient ratio.[79]

Apart from patient care, nurses are also entrusted to perform other functions like that of the dietician, in charge of arranging accessories and a social worker. Moreover it is the nurses who report to the doctor and to the patients' relations about the progress made by the patients. The actual working hour allotted to the nurses is divided among clerical (keeping records of patients admitted and patients discharged) and the patient care duties. Moreover in most cases nurses are not supported by the Class IV staff of the hospital. Their non-cooperation causes great hindrances for them to perform the patient care duties.[80]

The government has openly confessed and identified the crisis faced by the health sector. In the 44th National Conference of the Associations of Physicians held in Kolkata in 1989, the then chief minister Jyoti Basu in his inaugural speech admitted the failure of the state to provide proper healthcare to its population. He pointed out that the breakdown of the state-funded healthcare infrastructure was mainly due to the shortage of funds. As an alternative proposal, he had invited the private sector in healthcare to share the responsibility. The private sector should also think of investing in and delivering healthcare to its population at large. Basu suggested that each private hospital should treat 20/30 patients free of cost.[81]

Keeping aside these general loopholes of the healthcare infrastructure in the decades following Independence, the services provided by the government hospitals were miserable.

Section II

A substantial part of the private healthcare sector[82] existed between 1947 and the pre-liberalization era. But neither in India, nor in most other developing countries, was there any governmental policy directed towards the promotion of private healthcare. It is only in the recent past that the policies promoted by the World Bank and other international organizations have placed a high priority upon the increasing role of this sector, especially in the developing countries.[83]

In most developing countries, even a few decades back, the government was viewed as the sole player in the healthcare sector. The International Conference on Primary Health Care, Alma Ata, in 1978, strongly reaffirmed that health was a fundamental human right and that the attainment of the highest possible level of health was a most important worldwide social goal whose realization required active inputs from many other social and economic sectors in addition to the health sector. The primary position of the government, at least in the policymakers' eyes, was confirmed by the influential Alma Ata declaration, which viewed the government as the major vehicle for improvement in people's health status.[84] However, a great deal has been researched and written about the performance of the public healthcare providers but similar knowledge on the private health sector has only begun to emerge over the last few years.[85]

Jesani and Anantharam[86] have correctly pointed out that the private sector and the relevance of privatization policies in the healthcare services are perhaps the least studied areas in our country. Notwithstanding all statements made in our plan documents and policy statements, it is evident that in healthcare it is the private sector rather than the public sector which occupies a predominant place. According to these two scholars mentioned above, over 80 per cent of doctors of all systems of medicine taken together and almost an equal proportion of the healthcare expenditure in our country are accounted for by the private sector. It is therefore amply clear that the policy of turning a blind eye to the private healthcare sector has created a monster which is eating away a big chunk of India's valuable resources.[87]

The idea of calling upon private capital for financing healthcare was first clearly articulated in the document 'Financing Health Care: An Agenda for Reform' (World Bank 1987), which set the policy agenda for the late 1980s.[88] However, the importance of the private health sector was recognized properly only after the publication of the *World Development Report 1993: Investing in Health*.[89] This was actually a manifestation of the trend towards international mobilization around the theme of a smaller role for the government in healthcare.

Global policymakers have tended to recognize the WDR 1993 as the 'starting point' for recognizing the private healthcare sector as a major component of health services. What is significant is that private healthcare which had existed in the form of small nursing homes and clinics (in the early years after Independence, in the case of India) was overlooked completely by international agencies and global policymakers. The pressure from various international bodies to reduce the level of government involvement in healthcare and promote the private sector accelerated its growth. Interestingly, the recommendations made in the reports to strengthen the drive towards privatization of the healthcare delivery services have a very weak information base about the functioning of existing private healthcare providers and the quality and efficiency of the services offered by them. Bennett, McPake and Mills[90] have shown that, in response to criticisms levelled at it, the arguments in favour of the private sector have become increasingly sophisticated. Instead of simply advocating a greater role for private providers, more complex strategies have emerged such as creating competition between providers through competitive contracting,[91] expanding access to services through subsidizing private providers and encouraging the more wealthy to use private providers so that government resources can be better targeted on the poor. But the empirical knowledge for policymaking is still very limited in this area.

Let us return to the fact that private healthcare existed substantially prior to globalization. In the pre-globalization-liberalization era, private healthcare was confined almost entirely to *secondary level* healthcare. Post-reform policies or more precisely *globalization* provided the platform whereby private players were allowed large-scale entry into *tertiary level* healthcare. And herein lies the significance of post-liberalization privatization. Since tertiary level healthcare involves multispecialty hospitals, privatization in this domain implies a large-scale influx of corporate capital. Thus as opposed to pre-liberalization private healthcare, post-liberalization privatization is in essence corporatization. From now on, healthcare would flaunt itself quite unabashedly as a purely business proposition where the profits would mostly come from the upwardly mobile social strata, in place of the nationalist and leftist image of healthcare as a service for all the people.

In a recent study, Baru has pointed out that the private sector is structurally plural and hierarchical in its organization. The primary level of care is dominated by individual practitioners in rural and urban areas who can be classified as those who are formally and informally trained across systems of medicine. The secondary level is occupied by small and medium nursing homes promoted by a single owner or partnership, mostly among doctors. A large proportion of the private sector continues to be dominated by independent practitioners, formal and informal, followed by small and medium enterprises and a small segment which is private and public limited. The secondary level of care in the private sector consists of small and medium nursing homes that are promoted by single owners or partners, mostly doctors. These nursing homes are located in urban, semi-urban and rural areas. Across income quintiles, these nursing homes are being used for outpatient and inpatient services.[92]

It is necessary to mention that the private nursing homes, in the early period after Independence, did not mushroom due to any global drive towards privatization. Nor was it due to so much dismal performance of the public sector. The real impetus towards setting up nursing homes sprang from a number of causes. First and foremost was the need, felt by somewhat affluent middle-class families, of getting more *personalised* care than was possible in government health establishments. Secondly, there was among physicians a set of entrepreneurs who felt the drive to address this need. But, the whole thing operated at a rather small scale. The nursing home was in many ways an extension of the doctor's private practice. Hence, the nursing homes often had a personal touch; sometimes the patients' meals would be cooked by the doctor's wife or at least the cooking supervised by her. This scenario was to change radically in the 1990s when healthcare-acquired industrial proportions.

Under the West Bengal Clinical Establishments Act of 1950, it is mandatory for all nursing homes to get registered. However, the list of registered nursing homes available with the state health department does not show their date of establishment. Instead, it shows the date of renewal of the registration. As a result, it is difficult to have an idea of the growth of private nursing homes over the years. There is also the absence of crucial information on a large number of establishments.

The West Bengal Clinical Establishment Act of 1950 was an Act to introduce the system of registration and licencing in respect of the clinical establishment. The statements and objectives of the Act were available in the proceedings of the meetings of the West Bengal Legislative Assembly held on 29 September 1950 and the Act came into force on 15 February 1952. It has clarified 'clinical establishment' as any nursing home, physical therapy establishment, clinical laboratory, hospital, dispensary (with bed) medical camp, medical clinic, medical institution of analogous establishment, by whatever name called. According to this Act, 'maternity home' means where women are usually (received or accommodated or both) for the purpose of confinement and ante-natal and post-natal care in connection with childbirth. While 'nursing home' is an establishment where persons suffering from illness, injury or infirmity whether of body or mind are usually for the purpose of nursing and treatment and includes maternity homes. No person can keep or carry a medical establishment without being registered in respect of a licence granted therefore. West Bengal Clinical Establishment Act 1950 has clarified different clauses regarding the application for getting registered under this Act. It has also pointed out the rules about the cancellation of the registration and licence of the 'clinical establishments'.[93]

The Private Health Sector: History of Small Nursing Homes and Private Hospitals in Kolkata after Independence

There is a serious paucity of data regarding the nature or even size of the private health sector. The government documents have not recorded its growth and there seems to be almost deliberate silence on documenting the rise of the private health sector.

However, the classification of hospitals on the basis of ownership pattern in *Health on the March* does speak of a private sector. But this 'private sector' does not represent the nursing homes that grew up in the decades after Independence. On the other hand, according to the 1962 issue of the *Health on the March*,[94] we come across two categories of private hospitals:

(i) Private aided
(ii) Private non-aided

We have noted that in 1962, the number of hospitals and hospital beds under 'private aided category' were 23 and 3,146, respectively, while the corresponding figures under the private non-aided category were only 6 and 290. In 1963,[95] the 'private aided' category had been replaced by 'state-aided' hospitals and the number of such hospitals had been slightly reduced to 22 and the number of beds to 3,047. From 1972, the 'private aided' category generally came to signify philanthropic organizations (including missionary efforts). With some alteration of the basis of calculating the number of hospitals and hospital beds, again from 1979,[96] there had been the re-appearance of the 'private aided' category. However, the category 'private non-aided' continued to remain unclear.

But it is beyond doubt that neither the 'private aided' nor the 'private non-aided' category represented the *nursing homes of Calcutta.*

Not a single government document makes any reference to the existence of nursing homes in the city of Calcutta in the decades immediately following Independence.

However, *Swasthya Dwipika,*[97] in an editorial in its December 1967 issue, while describing the healthcare infrastructure in Calcutta, devoted just a single sentence mentioning that Calcutta had 50/60 private nursing homes. Discussions with physicians who were active during the 1960s indicate that the above estimate is possibly an exaggeration and the actual number would not have been more than 40.

Sections of the medical establishment in the 1950s were not comfortable with the fast growth of the nursing homes in the city. This is revealed in the editorial of JIMA in its May 1952 issue, which also recorded that Calcutta had witnessed the cropping up of a large number of 'bath and massage clinics'.[98]

> In the post-Independence period private nursing homes started mushrooming in a limited way. Of late, in the city of Calcutta large numbers of bath and massage clinics have cropped up whose main objective appears to be to dupe the unsophisticated and earn a living out of him. Most of these establishments are run in a most clandestine fashion and there have been several raids by the local police to put a stop to this growing menace. But the existing law was found to be insufficient to cope with the situation.[99]
>
> While we agree that the so-called massage and bath clinics were doing more harm to the society than good and that preventive measures and definite control over these establishments were indispensably necessary, we do feel that these clinical laboratories and treatment centres run by doctors should be exempted from the operation of the Clinical Establishments Act recently introduced in this province and urge upon the Government to keep such establishments outside the scope of this Act.[100]

Initially, the patients seemed to be somewhat uncomfortable with private medical establishments and did not have any clear idea about these.[101] Private nursing homes were not accepted wholeheartedly. This sector was confined to an entirely different sphere or a space from which the common people were debarred. Its service was meant for a particular section that had the capacity to afford cleaner environment, more privacy and personalized attention, different from that available in the overcrowded and unsanitized public hospitals.

As there is a lack of historical records in this regard, I have depended on the oral sources – interviews with medical personnel of the city – to weave the story of the growth of nursing homes in Calcutta. This survey is based entirely on interviews with the physicians, managers or administrators and sometimes with the nurses and attendants of the nursing homes. The nursing homes that are unevenly distributed all over Kolkata were chosen on a random basis.

It needs to be stressed here that the growth and development of the private healthcare sector, particularly from the late 1940s to the mid-1980s, may not be associated with:

(i) Decline of public hospitals
(ii) Initiatives on behalf of the government to invite private capital in healthcare
(iii) Impact of the forces of globalization, converting healthcare to a purchasable commodity
(iv) A public–private partnership project

All those, to varying extent, became operative from the late 1990s.

Certain obvious limitations cropped up in the process of interviewing. Most often, we found that people gave the answer that they felt the interviewer wanted them to give. There are also disparities as far as the opinions are concerned because often they differ on the facts. Ann Cartwright[102] has correctly pointed out that in this type of survey, the opinion given in response to specific questions are often so lightly held that they are better regarded as random whims. There are also tendencies to reduce complexities which sometimes lead to a kind of distortion.

Nevertheless, once we keep the above caveats in mind, the interviews become a valuable source of information. We have interviewed personnel from a total of 38 institutions – small and medium private nursing homes on the one hand and large private corporate hospitals on the other.

Emergence of the small nursing homes in Calcutta after Independence is a separate phenomenon which has no linkages with the general trend of the growth of the private healthcare that surfaced from the late 1970s.

The reasons behind the growth of nursing homes in the city are numerous. Since there is a dearth of documentary sources, we shall base our arguments on our conversations with the senior doctors and health activists who had witnessed the healthcare scenario following Independence.

The existence of private nursing homes can be traced back to the 1950s and 1960s. According to some estimates, well over half the available health services were being provided by the private sector even as early as the 1960s.[103] Indeed, as far as Kolkata is concerned, traces of small nursing homes (in terms of bed strength and services) could be found even from the early years of Independence. Recollecting the presence of private nursing homes in Kolkata, a senior resident narrated that in the early 1950s, the doctor entrepreneurs started very few nursing homes and these institutions mainly dealt with delivery cases.[104] The need for private nursing homes was not seriously felt by the patients and the concept of nursing homes as a separate healthcare organization did not take proper shape in their minds. They were satisfied with the services provided by the public hospitals and the doctor–patient relationship was not much commercialized. However, there was a general tendency among the patients to either consult one's family physician in his private chamber or visit the outpatient department (OPD) of a private hospital or charitable trust. It is not a recent development that most patients belonging to the below poverty line (BPL) category use the OPD of government hospitals.[105] According to *India Health Report*, more than half the available health services were being provided by the private sector as early as the 1950s.[106]

According to health activist Amal Bose,[107] the causes for the mushrooming of small nursing homes in Calcutta are many. The decade of 1947–1957 was a period of transition when the British model was predominant in healthcare structure. The colonial hangover was present in almost all aspects of life. He recollects that during this phase, in the northern parts of Calcutta a few nursing homes came up having the infrastructure of maternity homes. These were old-fashioned nursing homes where the Anglo-Indian community took admission for treatment. Sometimes they were founded by the missionaries. Some nursing homes were also established by young doctors who were trained abroad. These doctors after their return to India set up nursing homes on the model of the British healthcare institutes. In those days, the doctors were mostly appointed in public hospitals, but simultaneously they could also practise privately and set up nursing homes under their own supervision to expand their practice.

Between 1957 and 1967, there was large-scale urbanization and industrialization in Calcutta and its peripheral areas.[108] This led to the increasing population inflow into the city. Both the processes of urbanization and industrialization brought about different kinds of diseases. The public hospitals were already saturated with their patients, and the need for more healthcare organizations during this period gave rise to nursing homes.

Bose also points out that the period between 1967 and 1977 witnessed political turmoil and the Naxalite movement. The victims of political clashes and the injured Naxalites were often denied admission to public hospitals. A number of small nursing homes mushroomed during this period in different corners of the city as an alternative place for their treatment.

There was a large-scale development of the nursing homes between 1977 and 1987 when the Metro Transit System linked up several corners of the city. Population inflow in and around the peripheral areas and the rise of varied occupational groups along with their need for better healthcare posed a challenge to the existing healthcare system. The degeneration of the public hospitals had already set in and private healthcare mostly in the form of nursing homes and private hospitals had surfaced to satisfy the needs of the population at large.

Amal Bose has vividly narrated the story behind the transformation of Kolkata into a globalized metropolis from 1987 to 1997. New modes of urbanization like building highways and flyovers, utilizing the unused spaces for constructing residential complexes and investing private capital in every sphere characterized this phase. Increasing connectivity to the city boosted the population inflow and simultaneously generated the demand for sanitized space in healthcare. Thus Bose feels that in the latter part of the twentieth century, private healthcare no longer signified the small nursing homes. Their places were taken up by big corporate hospitals. He also mentions that the reduction in the size of the family increased the loss of tolerance and the manpower needed to take care of the hassles of treatment in public hospitals. This is one of the reasons which increased the demand for the private healthcare sector where one could get hassle-free services and treatment in lieu of money.

According to historian Ranjit Sen,[109] during the 1940s, 1950s and 1960s, people did not go to private healthcare centres. So, there was no effective demand for the establishment of nursing homes. Till then, the R.G. Kar Hospital,

Calcutta Medical College and P.G. Hospital served the population of the city at large. However, the Nilratan Sirkar Medical College and National Medical College were not so popular. These mainly served the east Calcutta population. The Sealdah railway station was crowded with refugees and middle-class Bengali patients. Nilratan Sirkar Medical College generally served the patients from north suburban areas and the National Medical College was utilized by the patients of south suburban areas. The Park Circus railway station acted as a communication halt for the south suburban masses. As a result, people from these areas never went to P.G. or R.G. Kar hospital for treatment. Prof. Sen also mentions that in the latter part of the 1940s, there was the Lake Camp Hospital. It mainly served the American soldiers and the well-off sections of the south Kolkata (Rashbehari Avenue, Chetla and New Alipore) population. Doctors of Lake Camp Hospital also practised in National Medical College, P.G. Hospital and Calcutta Medical College. As a result, there was no dearth of doctors in the public sector. He recollects that in 1959, his father Pabitra Sen (a retired meteorologist) was suffering from a perforated ulcer. This critical case was treated in P.G. Hospital where a medical board was set up under Dr Lalit Bannerjii and Dr Anjali Chatterjii. It is noteworthy that the latter, a woman physician, had been appointed on the board. Prof. Sen comments that even in late 1950s and early 1960s, the government hospitals had the best doctors and medical facilities for treating complicated cases.

Calcutta had to wait for another decade to witness the largescale mushrooming of small nursing homes. Prof. Sen observes that from the mid-1960s onwards the trend of going abroad either for higher education or for employment increased greatly. This resulted in the inflow of capital into the city, since the people who went overseas with jobs often sent remittances at home. At the same time, in the southern parts of Calcutta, there was an emergence of a comparatively affluent, enlightened and health-conscious section which was not satisfied with the situation in the public hospitals. The degeneration of the public hospitals had already surfaced during this period. Moreover, the huge refugee population (often affected by diseases) also put tremendous pressure on the infrastructure of the public hospitals. Educated and solvent families no longer wanted to admit their relatives to the congested government hospitals. Too much pressure of patients accelerated the process of deterioration of the quality of service. Thus, there was an increasing need for healthcare organizations where the affluent sections of the society could find comfort and better treatment.

Against this backdrop, Prof. Sen points out another factor responsible for the growth of nursing homes in Calcutta. During this time women were getting a higher education and coming out in large numbers for employment. This trend was mostly visible in south Calcutta where the women of the educated middle-class families preferred to be admitted for delivery either in Ramakrishna Mission Seva Pratishthan or in Matri Sadan near Tollygunge railway bridge at Sri Mohan Lane. From this time onwards gynaecological complications increased since women were increasingly coming out to the public spheres from their sheltered life. They were unused to the stress and tension of the outside world. Demand for female doctors increased and this period witnessed the emergence of small nursing homes which mainly served as maternity homes. There was already a considerable patient load on Ramakrishna Mission and Matri Sadan. So, an obvious demand arose for more private healthcare institutions with better treatment and updated technological support.

The new generation of doctors returning from the UK or USA, trained in new medical technologies, found the infrastructure of public hospitals unsuitable for their practice. Moreover, all the posts were saturated by senior physicians and the procedures of new recruitment and transfer were characterized by unhealthy politics and nepotism. The salaries in the government hospitals were also poor. As a result, these new generation doctors established nursing homes under their own supervision and created an atmosphere where they could practise and implement their new knowledge of medicine. In addition to this, bank financing started in a small way in the late 1960s. Private institutions started to grow up and some nursing homes were also established after taking loans from the banks.

With the gradual degeneration of the public hospitals, the middle class slowly moved away from public hospitals and shifted to nursing homes. This also increased the demand for the setting up of general nursing homes in the city.

Stalwart physicians in government hospitals had failed to create their replacements for the new generations. This resulted in a vacuum of quality doctors in public hospitals. The absorption of good doctors by the private nursing homes and hospitals (in the later half of the 1980s) increased the popularity of the private healthcare establishments.

A series of private hospitals emerged in the western parts of Calcutta. Alipore and New Alipore were inhabited by the upper-middle-class sections of the society. Woodlands and Belle Vue were their only places of treatment. But with the increasing population pressure, the need for private hospitals increased in this region. Moreover, the Muslims of Budge Budge, Bata Nagar, Metiabruz and Khidderpore were no longer satisfied with the treatment in the P.G. Hospital. They needed a hospital nearby where they could go easily. This opportunity was taken up by the Kotharis and Birlas. Thus from the late 1970s there was the growth of Kothari, B.M. Birla and CMRI hospitals.

Prof. Sen also points out that the onslaught of lifestyle diseases created the need for specialized departments in private healthcare institutions. Till the 1980s, cardiac care units were not present in the private sector. B.M. Birla was the first private healthcare institution which developed specialized cardiac care units.

Dr Sudhir Ghosh[110] recalls that from the late 1960s onwards the services of the public hospitals had already started deteriorating due to excessive population pressure. In the initial stage, the private healthcare sector meant only maternity homes and small nursing homes where gynaecological cases and minor surgeries were undertaken. For complicated diseases and surgeries, people still utilized the services of the public hospitals. However, in course of time general nursing homes also emerged in Kolkata. The city had to wait for two more decades to witness the growth of private and corporate hospitals. Dr Ghosh feels that the small nursing homes were for those people who were dissatisfied with the services of the public hospitals but could not afford to admit their patients in Belle Vue and Woodlands.

However, the growth of the nursing homes in this phase was not a response to the failure of the public healthcare infrastructure. It was not even the answer to the shrinking responsibilities of the welfare state which was promoting the private healthcare sector to gain a solid footing. The rise of the private healthcare sector in this span of time was a separate and unique phenomenon.

The interviewed institutions are as follows.

Nursing homes established in the late 1940s and 1950s:

- Mother's Home (Exact date not Known, early years of the 1940s)
- East End Nursing Home Pvt. Ltd (1949)
- North Calcutta Nursing Home (1950)
- Citizen's Nursing Home Pvt. Ltd (1952)
- East End Nursing Home (1959)
- Woodlands Medical Centre (1944)

Nursing homes established in the 1960s

- Southern Nursing Home (1962)
- Calcutta Maternity and Nursing Home (1963)
- Northland Nursing Home (1964)
- Park Site Nursing Home (1968)
- Eveland Nursing Home & Infertility Clinic (1969)
- Dr B.N. Bose Memorial Clinic, Apollo Nursing Home (1969)
- Belle Vue Clinic (1969)

Nursing homes established in the 1970s

- Lion's Orthopaedic Hospital & Research Centre (1970)
- Sri Aurobindo Seva Kendra (SASK) (1971)
- United Nursing Home (early years of 1970s, exact date is not known)
- St Mary's Nursing Home Pvt. Ltd (1974)
- Repose Clinic & Research Centre Pvt. Ltd (1975)
- Bright Nursing Home (1975)
- Lake View Nursing Home (1975)
- Dreamland Nursing Home (1976)

Nursing homes established in the 1980s

- Prince Nursing Home (1982/83)
- Good Hope Nursing Home (Early years of 1980s, exact date not known)
- Swiss Park Nursing Home (1984)
- South Kolkata Clinic (1984)
- Udayan Nursing Home & Investigation Complex (1984)

- Orchid Nursing Home (1985)
- Dr Mina Mazumdar Seba Mandir Pvt. Ltd (1988)

Nursing homes established in the 1990s

- Rameswara Nursing Home (1991)
- Peerless Hospital and B.K. Roy Research Centre (1993)
- Care Hospital (1993/94)
- Microlap (1996)
- Zenith Point (1996)
- Paramount Nursing Home Pvt. Ltd (1996)
- Shee Medical Centre (1996)
- Advanced Medicare & Research Institute (AMRI) (1996)
- Cure Centre Nursing Home (1998)
- Five Point Micro Surgery Centre (1998)

In Table 3.6 we present a scenario of these nursing homes constructed on the basis of information retrieved from the interviews.

Interviews with some of the senior physicians reveal that the nursing homes were very few in number in the next two decades following Independence. The small nursing homes were mostly maternity clinics undertaking delivery cases. These nursing homes were generally established by an individual doctor with some specialization. A doctor under his or her own supervision established a nursing home in one's own house or in a rental house to provide 'service' to the community at large. The doctor-entrepreneur was often also attached to a government hospital. Sometimes the nursing homes were set up in partnership by two or more doctors. Unlike the present day, corporate bodies and private limited companies were seldom present as investors in healthcare. Non-medical persons rarely invested in the sector. Generally speaking, most of the nursing homes were very small, having 10 to 15 beds. The services or facilities provided were also very limited.

Minor surgeries in gynaecology, general surgeries of the gall bladder, appendix and hernia, as well as ophthalmologic surgeries were undertaken. Actually, the infrastructure in these nursing homes was generally limited and they could never offer major surgical services. Before the establishment of private hospitals (with the notable exception of Woodlands and Belle Vue), people generally flocked to government hospitals for major surgeries and complicated cases.

The nursing homes established in the 1940s and 1950s are now in a decaying state. The phenomena of individual doctors acting as entrepreneurs setting up nursing homes and the latter being mainly maternity centres continued in the 1960s. However, this period also witnessed the mushrooming of small nursing homes undertaking only gynaecological and obstetric cases.

Only a few of the early institutions like the Northland Nursing Home (initially a maternity home, later transformed into a general nursing home) have been able

Table 3.6 Nursing Homes and Private Hospitals in Kolkata from the mid-1940s to the 1990s: A Generalized Overview[111]

Date of establishment	Institution	Type of Accommodation	Source of Funds	Bed Strength	Staff Strength	Services	Expansion over the Years	Utilization Pattern[112]	Situation at Present
Exact date not known. Roughly 60 years old at the time of interview	**Mother's Home**	Rented house	Personal funds of Dr Bimal Chakraborty	5	8 (including 1 RMO)	Mostly gynaecological cases, other minor surgeries are also undertaken	No substantial expansion has taken place	Then: Local, upper middle class patients. Now: Urban poor, refused admission by government hospital for lack of beds.	Almost declined
1949	**East End Nursing Home Pvt. Ltd**	Rented house	A group of doctors invested their personal savings	12	10–12 (including 1 RMO)	Mostly gynaecological cases, other minor surgeries are also undertaken	No expansion of any service over time	Then: Upper-middle-class patients from the posh south Calcutta. Now: Patients residing in the slums of Park Circus area.	Almost in a state of decay
1950	**North Calcutta Nursing Home**	Situated in an old house in North Kolkata	Dr Asru Kumar Roy and Dr A.N. Dhole. Both of them invested their personal funds	14	18	Mostly gynaecological cases are treated. Other surgical cases like orthopaedic, eye, ENT, etc., are also undertaken	Increase in number of beds, introduction of other treatments along with gynaecological cases	Then: Upper middle-class and middle class. Now: No substantial change in patient profile.	Shut down
1952	**Citizen's Nursing Home Pvt. Ltd**	Rented house	Dr S.K. Mitra's personal funds	7	10.	Initially a maternity home, later other cases are attended to	Increase in the number of beds, treatment of other ailments	Then: Upper middle class from the adjoining areas. Now: Only poor people come for treatment.	Almost decaying
1959	**East End Nursing Home**	Rented house	Personal funds of Dr S K. Sur Ray	5	7	All kinds of obstetric and gynaecological cases	No expansion in any of the services	Then: Upper middle class and middle class of the city. Now: Lower middle class of the surrounding areas.	Almost in a state of decay

(Continued)

Table 3.6 (Continued)

Date of establishment	Institution	Type of Accommodation	Source of Funds	Bed Strength	Staff Strength	Services	Expansion over the Years	Utilization Pattern[112]	Situation at Present
1944	**Woodlands Medical Centre** (Woodlands Nursing Home)[113]	Own building	Donation by corporate members	230	125	All kinds of services, including super-specialized departments	Increase in the number of beds and diversification of various services	Then: Upwardly mobile sections. Now: Upwardly mobile and middle-class patients.	Running successfully
1962	**Southern Nursing Home**	Located in the house of Dr S.P. Ghosh	Personal funds of Dr S.P. Ghosh	26	Inadequate information	Initially treated gynaecological cases, now has other specialized departments	Along with increase in the number of beds, ICCU, ambulance, diagnostic services and other departments have been introduced	No substantial change in patient profile. Middle-class patients generally come for treatment.	Running successfully
1963	**Calcutta Maternity and Nursing Home**	Rented floor at top of a cinema hall (Radha Cinema)	Adequate information not available	6	7	Minor surgeries, especially gynaecological cases are undertaken	No expansion over the years	Patients from the lower economic level come for treatment. No change in patient profile.	In a decaying state
1964	**Northland Nursing Home**	A spacious rented building	Dr S. K. Roy's personal funds	14	40	Generally all types of surgeries are undertaken. Initially, cardiac and ophthalmologic surgeries were also performed. But cardiac patients are not	No substantial expansion. Five beds were converted to ICU/ITTU beds in 1999	No substantial change in patient profile. Patients from both high and middle-income groups come for treatment. Low-income group patients are fewer in number	Though the initial glory has faded, it is running successfully

1968	**Park Site Nursing Home**	Rented house	Personal investments of the five partners	19	10	Used to undertake gynaecological and obstetric surgeries initially. But in course of time, general surgeries were also undertaken	Number of beds increased from 10 to 19 with the rising patient pressure. But again reduced to 10	Then: Patients from high-income group. Now: Patients include the urban poor and underprivileged rural people.	Surviving in a break-even condition
1969	**Eveland Nursing Home & Infertility Clinic**	The nursing home was initially started in a rented house in, 2, Southern Avenue with only one bed. Gradually the bed strength increased to 9. In early 1980s, the present house which was initially a two-storied building with a pond was bought and the reconstructions started four years later. A multi-storied building was constructed for setting up the nursing home.	The professional income of Dr Rathin Ghosh along with some loans	24	100	The nursing home provides multiple services apart from the in-patient department (special emphasis on gynaecological cases)	Substantial expansion has taken place	Then: Patients from higher income group. Now: Lower middle class and even economically challenged sections.	Shut down
1969	**Dr B.N. Bose Memorial Clinic, Apollo Nursing Home**	Started in Dr Bose's own house	Personal investments of Dr Bose and his ancestral inheritances were the chief sources of funds	4	More than 40 employees including 7/8 RMOs	General surgeries, orthopaedic cases, general medicine cases, gynaecological and paediatric cases are undertaken	Along with the increase in the number of beds, multiple services are also undertaken.	Then: Middle class, lower middle class and lower economic strata. Now: Affluent sections also visit this nursing home.	The nursing home is doing well at present

(Continued)

Table 3.6 (Continued)

Date of establishment	Institution	Type of Accommodation	Source of Funds	Bed Strength	Staff Strength	Services	Expansion over the Years	Utilization Pattern[12]	Situation at Present
1967	**Belle Vue Clinic**[114]	Own spacious building	Investments by the Birla group	72	More than 500	All kinds of services, including super-specialized departments	Substantial expansion in multiple services	No remarkable change in the profile of patients, who are mostly from the upper class of Kolkata.	Running successfully
1970	**Lion's Orthopaedic Hospital & Research Centre**	Lion's Orthopedic Hospital & Research Centre is a part of the International Federation of Lion's Club. The house and the adjacent land where the hospital is located belonged to the Murarka family. They donated their entire property to the hospital authority who has set up the hospital.	Donations by the Murarka family	20	30	Houses both outpatient and inpatient departments (including diagnostic services)	Inpatient department and other services were added later	Provides healthcare to the downtrodden people since inception.	Running successfully
1971	**Sri Aurobindo Seva Kendra (SASK)**	The stretch of land, where the nursing home stands, was given by K.M.C. in 1971 but the building was constructed in 1990. Initially, the nursing home was situated in 71 and 73 Jodhpur Park with minimum infrastructure	Economic Entrepreneurship Development Foundation (EEDF), a company investing in health, agriculture and engineering	150	Inadequate information	Offers a wide range of services and facilities.	Sub-sequent expansion has taken place since inception	Patients from different socio- economic backgrounds.	Running successfully

Year	Name	Building/Start	Source of funds			Services	Expansion	Patient profile	Status
Early 1970s (exact date not known)	**United Nursing Home**	Started in a leased house	Personal funds of Dr J. Chaudhuri	34	20	Undertakes all kinds of cases	No substantial expansion has taken place	Then: Affluent sections of the society. Now: Mainly urban poor.	Shut down
1974	**St. Mary's Nursing Home Pvt. Ltd**	The nursing home is located in a hundred year old residential house of the colonial period. The family of Dr A. K. Deb resided here from 1974 –2007. After the death of Dr Deb in June 2007 his son sold the nursing home to a business house. But the nursing home was in a rented house	Personal savings of Dr A. K. Deb	35	Adequate information not available	Undertakes all types of surgical cases	There has been no expansion	Then: Upwardly mobile sections. Now: The unprivileged sections who do not get admission in government hospitals.	Shut down
1975	**Repose Clinic & Research Centre Pvt. Ltd**	Purchased house	Personal funds of Dr Mayarani Ghosh	60	More than 150	Providing multiple services	Large-scale expansion has taken place	Mostly upper middle class and middle class patients.	Running in a good condition
1975	**Bright Nursing Home**	Set up in the residential building Dr Mrs Priti Chakraborty	Personal funds of Dr P. Chakraborty	12	15	Undertakes all types of surgical and medical cases	No expansion has taken place	No change in patient profile.	Shut down
1975	**Lake View Nursing Home**	The nursing home is located in Dr Roy Chowdhury's own house in South Kolkata. The ground floor and the third floor of the building were being utilized for nursing home purposes.	Personal investment of Dr Roy Chowdhury	10	15	Undertakes all types of surgical and medical cases	Only bed strength has increased	Then: upper-middle-class and middle-class patients. Now: Patients from the economically challenged sections	Shut down

(Continued)

Table 3.6 (Continued)

Date of establishment	Institution	Type of Accommodation	Source of Funds	Bed Strength	Staff Strength	Services	Expansion over the Years	Utilization Pattern[112]	Situation at Present
1976	**Dreamland Nursing Home**	Own house	Personal funds of Dr Sudhir Ghosh	60	110	Undertakes all types of surgical and medical cases. ICCU/ITU available	Expansion has taken place	Then: Both upwardly mobile section and patients from the lower economic strata come to Dreamland for treatment. Now: Upwardly mobile section of the society.	Running successfully
1982/83	**Prince Nursing Home**	Situated in a rented residential house	Personal savings and bank loan	9	16	General nursing home with only inpatient department	Only bed strength has increased	Then: Both upper-middle class and middle-class patients. Now: Very few patients.	Shut down
Early 1980s (exact date not known)	**Good Hope Nursing Home**	Own building	Personal funds of Dr Rakhi Bose	10	20	Undertakes all types of surgical and medical cases	Substantial expansion has taken place	Both upper-middle-class and middle-class patients.	Presently converted to Angel Nursing Home and it is running successfully
1984	**Swiss Park Nursing Home**	Located in the residential house of Dr S. Chatterji	Personal savings of Dr Chatterji and her husband	15	50 employees including two RMOs	Undertakes all types of surgical and medical cases	Substantial expansion has taken place	No remarkable change in patient profile.	Running successfully
1984	**South Calcutta Clinic**	Located in the residential building of the owners	Funds provided by the partners	50	62	Undertakes all types of surgical and medical cases	Number of beds increased, other services introduced	No major change in patient profile.	Not running with much success
1984	**Udayan Nursing Home & Investigation Complex**	Own building	Personal savings of Dr Bimal Ghosh	15	20	Provides multiple services	Expanded substantially	Middle-class and lower middle-class patients.	Almost decaying
1985	**Orchid Nursing Home**	Located in the residential house of Dr B. Chaudhuri	Personal savings of Dr Chaudhuri	18	Inadequate information	Undertakes a wide range of cases	No expansion has taken place	Then: Affluent sections used to visit the nursing home. Now: Patients hardly come.	Almost declining

Year	Name	Building	Source of funds			Services	Expansion	Patients	Status
1988	**Dr Mina Mazumdar Seba Mandir Pvt Ltd**	Located at the residence Dr Majumdar	Ancestral property	10	24	Undertakes different types of cases	No expansion	Middle-class and lower middle-class patients.	Shut down
1991	**Rameswara Nursing Home Private Limited**	Located in the four-storied building of Mr Ram Avatar	Investment by Mr Ram Avatar, a businessman selling mosquito nets	32	64	Undertakes all kinds of surgical and medical cases	Modern services available since inception	Upper middle-class and middle-class patients	Running in a good condition
1993	**Peerless Hospital and B.K. Roy Research Centre**	Own building	Peerless General Finance and Investment Company Limited	300	2,000	Multiple services provided	Substantial expansion has taken place	Patients from different socio- economic strata	Running successfully
1993-94	**Care Hospital**	Own building	A co-operative society comprising 64 doctors	28	25	Provides multiple services	No expansion due to lack of funds	Middle class and lower middle class patients.	Shut down
1996	**Microlap**	Own building	Dr Deepak Mukherjee's own funds and bank loan	60	60	General hospital having several specialized and super-specialized departments	Expanded rapidly	Patients belonging to higher- and middle-income groups.	Running successfully
1996	**Zenith Point**	Inadequate information	Personal funds of Dr Puroshattam Pal	15	Inadequate information	Gynaecological and obstetric cases are undertaken	No substantial expansion	Middle class and lower-middle-class patients.	Shut down
1996	**Paramount Nursing Home**	Own building	Personal investment Mr A. Nandy – a businessman	40	80	Attends to all types of cases and provides multiple services	Has modern facilities since inception	Mostly affluent sections of the society.	Running in a good condition
1996	**Shee Medical Centre**	Purchased house	Personal funds of Dr Indrajyoti Shee	10	10	General nursing home	Number of beds has increased	Middle-class patients.	Running successfully
1996	**Advanced Medicare & Research Institute (AMRI)**	Set up in the building of Niramoy Polyclinic (owned by Government of West Bengal)	Capital was invested by the Todi Group	160	Inadequate information	Provides all kinds of services. It also has a teaching and research section	Expanded substantially over the years	Upper middle class, middle-class lower middle-class patients.	Running successfully
1998	**Cure Centre Nursing Home**	Located in a five-storied building belonging to a lawyer	Investments by Indrajit Das, a contractor, and late A. Mandal, a decorator	30	70	Has only inpatient department with ICCU and ITU	No substantial expansion	Mostly middle-class patients.	Running successfully
1998	**Five Point Micro Surgery Centre**	Rented flat	Personal funds of Dr Arati Chakraborty	18	Inadequate information	Micro surgeries are undertaken	Expansion has taken place	Mostly middle-class patients.	Running in a good condition

to acclimatize themselves to cope with the changes in the private healthcare sector. They have degenerated for various reasons, mainly:

- Financial constraints.
- Lack of adequate infrastructure required for upgradation.
- The subsequent generation's lack of interest in medical profession.

Though the Northland Nursing Home has upgraded itself by introducing ICCU/ITUs, the inflow of patients has reduced to a large extent. The 12-bedded Southern Nursing Home dealing with gynaecological cases is also under severe constraint. However, the Relief Health Care and Research Private Limited, a company investing in healthcare, has taken over the nursing home and revived it from the crisis. Infusion of capital has infused new life into a degenerating organization. Park Site Nursing Home – a maternity home initially, later upgraded to a general nursing home – on the other hand, though in a decaying state, is still serving the community. The case of Eveland Nursing Home is also the same. Even the upgrading of services failed to control its decline. The rapid emergence of corporate hospitals in the peripheral areas brought about a setback for Eveland. The Apollo Nursing Home has revived from its period of crisis after a trust was formed to look after its financial part. The case of Belle Vue is an exception. Going against the general trend of private healthcare in the 1960s being identified with small nursing homes, it attracted the business magnates and the affluent sections of the society.

Established in the 1970s, Lake View Nursing Home, St Mary's, Bright Nursing Home and United Nursing Home have suffered a decline. But on the other hand, SASK, Dreamland and Repose Nursing Home are in a much better condition because they did not face financial pressure. However, in the case of SASK, the initial funding was provided by a private company and later the land for further expansion was given by the Calcutta Municipal Corporation. SASK has transformed into a multispecialty hospital from a small nursing home since it appropriately adapted itself to compete with the growing market of corporate healthcare service. Dreamland and Repose are running successfully since they have been able to modify themselves and expand their services with the rising demand.

The entry of non-medical personnel in healthcare for providing capital began slowly from the late 1970s. The nursing homes which had started their journey in this decade tried to upgrade themselves with the advent of the corporate hospitals in Calcutta. As a result, they have not suffered decay.

From the late 1980s onwards, the scenario started changing. The percentage of medical personnel investing in healthcare exhibited a sharp decline. Except Udayan, Orchid and Good Hope, the nursing homes of this period reviewed above were either a joint venture of a doctor and an entrepreneur or fully financed by non-medical persons. These nursing homes are also in a poor condition because they could not provide the corporate healthcare culture desired by most of the neo-elites of the globalized metropolis. In course of time it was also observed that the joint venture by a doctor and an entrepreneur could no longer bring about profit in the private healthcare institutions (e.g., Dr Mina Majumdar, South Calcutta Clinic and Prince Nursing Home). Though Good Hope is founded and managed by a doctor, it has upgraded its services and is running successfully. But other nursing homes of the 1980s are in a decaying state with the entry of big business houses, regional business groups and corporate capital.

This trend finally gathered momentum in the 1990s when AMRI, Peerless Hospital, Ruby General Hospital etc., emerged in the scenario of the private healthcare sector. Before that, a few big business houses had invested in healthcare in the 1980s, like in the case of B.M. Birla, Kothari and CMRI. But their presence was not dominant and they were only utilized by a particular section of the city people. Interestingly, in the nursing homes of the 1990s – Paramount, Cure Centre and Rameswara – investments were made by non-medical persons. There were decorators, contractors and businessmen among them, who had no connection with the healthcare sector. These nursing homes are running successfully and are competing with the private hospitals in the city. But presently the entire private healthcare sector, to a large extent, is in the hands of corporate capital.

However, in the 1990s, some small nursing homes were still coming up, such as Shee Medical Centre, Microlap, Zenith Point and Five Point Nursing Home. They are still functioning successfully in a period when the trend of establishing small nursing homes by an individual doctor has almost subsided. The question is whether these nursing homes coming up in the era of corporate healthcare culture will be able to survive in the long run. Will they have the same fate as the nursing homes that came up in the decades of the 1950s, 1960s and 1970s?

The entry of business groups in healthcare has undoubtedly transformed it into a profit-making industry where the place for socially committed doctors hardly exists. As a result, these nursing homes suffer a setback and are somewhat 'displaced' from their previous positions. A group of medical professionals cannot provide the amount of capital a business house can invest. Thus, the smaller nursing homes have failed to provide the expected services demanded by the neo-elite of globalized Kolkata. The insurance and cashless facilities have definitely increased the access to big hospitals for a particular section but this, on the other hand, totally devastated the small infrastructure nursing homes. So, in order to cope with these facilities, the smaller nursing homes are under severe financial crisis and sometimes on the verge of collapse.

Secondly, the doctors who had invested in healthcare in the 1960s and 1970s are no more active and due to lack of funds, they have failed to improve the infrastructure of their nursing homes. Owing to the absence of modern equipments, these nursing homes could not attract young doctors who were trained in state-of-the-art technologies. Nevertheless, in course of time, affordability has increased and people have become more health conscious. Status consciousness and love for comfort also played a crucial role behind their preference towards big private hospitals, which are highly sophisticated, well decorated, and more like 5-star hotels than healthcare institutions. As we have noted, the small nursing homes were mainly maternity homes, which in no way could provide multiple services under one roof.

A major shift has taken place as far as the utilization pattern is concerned. Patients who earlier went to public hospitals are now trying their best to get treated in private charitable (non-profit) hospitals like the Ramkrishna Mission Seva Pratishthan. The clientele of these charitable institutions are shifted towards small nursing homes, which were once utilized by the upwardly mobile sections of the society. The affluent social classes have moved out of these small nursing homes and are shifted towards big private hospitals. Cashless facilities have undoubtedly hastened this process of migration. At present, the urban poor and sometimes rural patients generally flock to government hospitals. Thus, a linkage in the investment pattern, growth process, nature of services and utilization pattern clearly justifies the changing face of the private healthcare sector in post-1947 Kolkata.

Presently, small and relatively inexpensive nursing homes cater to rural people who are able to afford a minimum level of private healthcare. As the public healthcare infrastructure has totally degenerated in the rural areas, people from these regions tend to flock to the city. The utterly poor make a beeline to the city's public hospitals, while those who may afford somewhat more try their luck in the small nursing homes. To them, getting admitted in a private nursing home in the city is also a mark of social status. Moreover, the urban population in the lower economic strata, having low-coverage medical insurance (Mediclaim), try these nursing homes, for the 'big' private hospitals are simply beyond their reach. Along with the increasing health awareness in almost all segments of the society, people have also come to believe that

- Public hospitals are no longer a better place for treatment.
- Quality treatment can be available only in the private nursing homes at a much higher price.

The small, once popular nursing homes are now catering to those who are not in a position to go to corporate hospitals but would not go to public hospitals either.

Notes

1 See R.V. Baru, *Factors Influencing Variations in Health Services: A Study of Selected Districts in Andhra Pradesh,* Unpublished M.Phil Dissertation, Jawaharlal Nehru University, 1987.
2 See Amrita Bagchi, "Public Health in Post Independence Kolkata", in the *Proceedings of the Indian History Congress,* 78th Session held in Jadavpur University, Kolkata, 28–30 December, 2017. ISSN 2249-1937 (2018), 1209–1215. (Hereafter cited as Bagchi, "Public Health in Post Independence Kolkata").
3 Ihtesham Kazi, "Environmental Factors Contributing to Malaria in Colonial Bengal", in *Medicine in India: A Historical Overview*, ed. Deepak Kumar (New Delhi: Tulika Books, 2001), 124.
4 J.C. Peterson, *Bengal District Gazetteers: Burdwan* (Calcutta: Bengal Secretariat Book Depot, 1910), 78, in Kumar, *Medicine in India A Historical Overview*, 129.
5 K.C. Ghosh, "Railway and Malaria LX11", March 1928, 169, in Kumar, *Medicine in India: A Historical Overview*, 129.
6 Arabinda Samanta, *Malarial Fever in Colonial Bengal 1820–1939: Social History of an Epidemic* (Kolkata: FIRMA KLM, 2002), 201.

7 Ibid.
8 Ibid.
9 *Samachar Darpan*, 27 April 1839, quoted by S.W. Goode, "Municipal Calcutta, its Institution in Their Origin and Growth", 232; Statistics compiled from Bengal Provincial Health Report 1919–1947, in Kabita Ray, *History of Public Health: Colonial Bengal 1921–1947* (Calcutta: K.P. Bagchi and Sons, 1998), 58–59.
10 Ibid., 345.
11 Ibid.
12 Ibid., 347.
13 Ibid., 345.
14 D.M. Moir, "Notes on the Origin of the Old Presidency General Hospital Calcutta", *Bengal Past and Present* 109, Part 1–2, no. 208–209 (1990): 122–34.
15 *Journal of Indian Medical Association* (JIMA), Supplement, Vol. XV111, No. 2 (Calcutta: 1948), XV11 (Hereafter cited as JIMA, supplement, Vol. XV111, No. 2).
16 Ibid.
17 Ibid.
18 Ibid.
19 Roger Jeffrey, *Politics of Health in India* (California: University of California Press, 1988), 51. For the details of Native Medical Institution, see Poonam Bala, *Imperialism and Medicine in Bengal: A Socio-Historical Perspective* (Sage Publications, 1991); Samita Sen and Anirban Das, "A History of the Calcutta Medical College and Hospital, 1835–1936", in *History of Science, Philosophy and Culture in Indian Civilization*, xv, *Science and Modern India: An Institutional History, c 1784–c 1947*, ed. Uma Dasgupta (Center for Studies in Civilizations, 2011); Biswamaoy Pati and Mark Harrison, *Health Medicine and Empire Perspectives on Colonial Medicine* (New Delhi: OUP, 2001), 37–87; D.G. Crawford, "Notes on the Early Hospitals of Calcutta", *Indian Medical Gazette* 38, no. 1 (1903).
20 JIMA, supplement, Vol. XV111, No. 2.
21 Ibid.
22 Ibid.
23 Ibid.
24 Ibid.
25 Ibid.
26 Ibid.
27 Ibid.
28 Ibid.
29 David Arnold, *Colonizing the Body: State Medicine and Epidemic Disease in Nineteenth Century India* (Berkeley: University of California Press, 1993); Roy Porter, *Health for Sale: Quackery in England, 1660–1850* (Manchester: Manchester University Press, 1989); Projit Bihari Mukharji, *Nationalizing the Body: The Medical Market, Print and Daktari Medicine* (New York: Anthem Press, 2009); Madhuri Sharma, *Indigenous and Western Medicine in Colonial India, Culture and Environment in South Asia* (New Delhi: Foundation Books, 2012) and Rachel Berger, *Ayurveda Made Modern: Political Histories of Indigenous Medicine in North India, 1900–1955*. Cambridge Imperial and Post-colonial Studies Series (New York: Palgrave Macmillan, 2013); Ratnabir Guha, "Native Bodies, Medical Market and 'Conflicting' Medical 'Systems': Venereal Diseases and the 'Vernacularisation' of Western Medical Knowledge in Colonial Bengal", *Presidency Historical Review* 1, no. 1 (March 13, 2015): 11–18.
30 For details on dispensaries see Projit Bihari Mukharji, "Structuring Plurality: Locality, Caste, Class and Ethnicity in Nineteenth-Century Bengali Dispensaries", *Health and History* 9, no. 1 (Australian and New Zealand Society of the History of Medicine, 2007); Christian Hochmuth, "Patterns of Medical Culture in Colonial Bengal, 1835–1880", *Bulletin of the History of Medicine* 80 (2006): 39–72.

31 AnjanBera, edited and compiled, *The Nation*, 8 November 1948, quoted in *Interpreting a Nation: Selections from Sarat Chandra Bose's The Nation* (Calcutta: Netaji Institute for Asian Studies, 2001), 67.
32 Ibid., 67.
33 Ibid., 68.
34 Ibid., 69.
35 Ibid., 70.
36 Ibid., 71.
37 Ibid.
38 Imrana Qadeer, "Health Services System in India: An Expression of Socio-Economic Inequalities", *Social Action* 35 (July–September 1985): 204.
39 Jean Drez and Amartya Sen, *India: Development and Participation* (New Delhi: Oxford University Press, 2002), 200–202.
40 See Chapter I of the book for details.
41 Presidential Address by Dr A.K. Basu at the 13th Bengal Provincial Medical Conference held in Midnapore on 7 and 8 November 1953, in *Journal of Indian Medical Association (JIMA)* xxiii, no. 5 (February 1954): 224.
42 Monidip Chatterjee, "Town Planning in Calcutta, Past, Present and Future", in *Calcutta: The Living City, The Present and Future*, vol. II, ed. Sukanta Chaudhuri (Calcutta: Oxford University Press, 1990) (Hereafter cited as Chaudhuri, *Calcutta: The Living City*), 142.
43 Ibid., 142.
44 Ibid., 143.
45 Raghab Bandopadhyay, "The Inheritors: Slum and Pavement Life in Calcutta", in Chaudhuri, *Calcutta: The Living City*, 78.
46 Ibid., 79.
47 Ibid., 82.
48 Ibid., 182.
49 See Bagchi, "Public Health in Post Independence Kolkata".
50 Ibid., 175.
51 Presidential Address by Dr A.K. Basu at the 13th Bengal Provincial Medical Conference at Midnapore, held on 7 and 8 November 1953, published in *Journal of Indian Medical Association* XX111, no. 5 (February 1954): 224.
52 Ibid.
53 Presidential Address by Dr A.C. Ukil, published in *Journal of Indian Medical Association* 26, no. 5 (March 1956): 174.
54 "*Blood Test e Malaria Virus Paowa Gechhe*". (Malaria Virus detected in blood test)', *Anandabazaar Patrika*, October 30, 1967.
55 "*Malaria: Prasthan o Prabesh* (Malaria: Exit and Entry)", *Anadabazaar Patrika*, November 12, 1967. This report narrated that long 67 years back, in 1900, preventive measures were first taken to control malaria outbreak. The same year, Malaria Commission of the Royal Society of England came to India to understand the situation of the epidemic. This commission for the first time stated that malaria was a National Problem of India. Another survey revealed that in 1935, more than 10 crore people were affected by malaria, of whom about 10 lakh died. In 1964, the Health Survey and Development Committee formulated a Health Action Plan to combat the disease. In 1946-47, Delhi, Bombay, Mysore and Uttar Pradesh also undertook the task to formulate the Pilot Action Plan. Surprisingly, though there were serious doubts regarding the success of these attempts, by 1952 it was observed that more than 3 crore people had responded to the preventive measures taken by the state.
56 "*Choleray 39 jon akranto* (39 people *infected by cholera*)" *Anandabazaar Patrika*, May 3, 1967.
57 *Health on the March* (various years).
58 Ibid.

59 Ibid.
60 Ibid.
61 Presidential Address by Dr B.P. Trivedi at the XVII Bengal Provincial Medical Conference, Bishnupur, 1958, published in *Journal of Indian Medical Association,* (Supplement), 3, no. 7 (October 1958),: 302.
62 *Health on the March* (1962).
63 *Health on the March* (1972).
64 See chapters, "The Demography of Calcutta" and "Calcutta's Environment", in *Calcutta: The Living City, The Present and Future*, vol. II, ed. Sukanta Chaudhuri (Calcutta: Oxford University Press, 1990).
65 *"National Medicalke sarkari niyantrane anar prastab"* (Proposal to bring National Medical under government control)', *Anandabazaar Patrika*, 3 May 1967; *"National Medical College-e gherao abyahata"* (Gherao continues in National Medical College), *Anandabazaar Patrika*, 14 May 1967; *"Chittaranjan Seba Sadan o Jatiyakaran"* (Nationalization of Chittaranjan Seva Sadan), *Anandabazaar Patrika*, 22 May 1967; *"Sarkari Parichalanay National Medical o Chittaranjan Hospital"* (National Medical and Chittaranjan Hospital under government management), *Anandabazaar Patrika*, 23 May 1967.
66 *"National Medical College: Kartripaksher Baktabya"* (National Medical College: Opinion of the Authorities), *Anandabazaar Patrika*, 7 June 1967.
67 *"National Medicale Ordinanace Balabat"* (Ordinance enforced in National Medical), *Anandabazaar Patrika*, 10 June 1967.
68 *"Towards Better Health in West Bengal"* (Progress since 1947) (Department of Health, Government of West Bengal, 1962).
69 Mani Kumar Chhetri, *Doctor*, Subhamoy Chatterjee and Nilanjan Dutta, ed., (Kolkata: Critical Care and Medical Education Trust, 2019).
70 Ibid.
71 Ibid.
72 Gaur Sen, *"Sahar Kolkatar Katha"*, *Swasthya Dwipika*, No. 12, Aghrayan-Paush 1374 (December 1967): 783–85.
73 Ibid.
74 *Health on the March* (various years).
75 Biswanath Paria, *An Appeal* (Calcutta: Medical Service Centre, 1985), 5. Also see *Swastha Bikshan,* January 2007.
76 Ibid., 11. Also see *Swastha Bikshan,* January 2007.
77 Molly Chattopadhyay, *Occupational Socialisation: A Study of Hospital Nurses* (Calcutta: Sarat Book House, 1993), 84–87.
78 Ibid.
79 Ibid.
80 Ibid.
81 *"Rajya sab pareni, tai prayojan besarkari haspataler"* (The s*tate has failed, so private hospitals are needed*), *Anandabazar Patrika*, 20 January 1989.
82 This category is referred as 'cottage industry' by Rama V. Baru. For details see Chapter 1.
83 Sara Bennet, Barbara McPake, and Anne Mills, "The Public/Private Mix Debate in Health Care", in *Private Health Providers in Developing Countries: Serving the Public Interest?,* ed. Sara Bennet, Barbara McPake, and Anne Mills (London: Zed Books, 1997), 1.
84 World Health Organization, *Primary Health Care: Report of the International Conference on Primary Health Care*, Alma Ata, USSR, 6-12, September 1978 (Geneva: WHO, 1979).
85 Barbara McPake, "The Role of Private Sector in Health Service Provision", in *Private Health Providers in Developing Countries: Serving the Public Interest?,* ed. Sara Bennet, Barbara McPake, and Anne Mills, 21.

86   A. Jesani and S. Anantharam, *Private Sector and Privatisation in the Health Care Service* (Bombay: FRCH, 1993), 1.

87   Ibid.

88   Sara Bennet, Barbara McPake, and Anne Mills, "The Public/Private Mix Debate in Health Care", 2.

89   World Bank, *World Development Report 1993 – Investing in Health* (New York: Oxford University Press, 1993).

90   Ibid., 2.

91   World Bank, *World Development Report 1993 – Investing in Health* (New York: Oxford University Press, 1993).

92   Rama V. Baru, "Medical Industrial Complex: Trends in Corporatization of Health Services", in *Equity and Access: Health Care Studies in India*, ed. Purendra Prasad and Amar Jessani (New Delhi: OUP, 2018), 79. For details of definition and classification of private health care sector see., *India Health Report*, ed. Mishra, Chatterjee, Rao (New Delhi: Oxford University Press, 2003), Anant Phadke, *Private Medical Sector in India* (Bombay: FRCH, 1994), Mohan Rao, "The State of Health in India", *South Asian Journal: Indo-Pak Dialogue*, October-December 2006, Ramesh Bhat, "The Private Health Care Sector in India", in *Paying for India's Health Care*, ed. Berman and Khan (New Delhi: Sage Publications, 1993), Alok Mukhopadhyay, ed. *Report of the Independent Commission on Health in India* (New Delhi: Voluntary Health Associations of India, 1997).

93   West Bengal Clinical Establishment Act 1950.

94   *Health on the March* (1962).

95   *Health on the March* (1963).

96   *Health on the March* (1973).

97   Gaur Sen, "Sahar Kolkatar Katha", *Swasthya Dwipika,* No. 12, Agrahayan–Paush 1374 (December 1967): 783–85.

98   JIMA, No. 8, May 1952, 371.

99   Ibid.

100 Ibid.

101 Interview with Ranjit Sen Calcutta University on 27.09.2007.

102 Ann Cartwright, *Human Relations and Hospital Care* (London: Routledge and Kegan Paul Limited, 1964), 64.

103 Rama V. Baru, *Private Health Care in India. Social Characteristics and Trends* (New Delhi: Sage Publications, 1998), 51.

104 Interview with Prof. Ranjit Sen at Calcutta University on 27.09.2007.

105 I made this observation from the interviews which I have conducted in private nursing homes at Kolkata and in Calcutta Medical College and Hospital in the entire course of my study.

106 Foreword by D.R. Gwatkin to Ramesh Bhat, *Private and Public Mix in Health Care in India* (Ahmedabad: IIM, 1995), In *India Health Report*, 102.

107 Interviewed on 08.05.2006.

108 See Amiya Kumar Bagchi, "Studies on the Economy of West Bengal since Independence", Basabi Bhattacharya, "Urbanisation and Human Development in West Bengal: A District Level Study and Comparison with Inter-State Variation", and Pabitra Giri, "Urbanisation in West Bengal, 1951–1991", *Economic and Political Weekly* (21 November 1998).

109 Professor of Islamic History and Culture, University of Calcutta, interviewed on 20.08.2007.

110 Dr Sudhir Ghosh is the founder and owner of Dreamland Nursing Home. He was interviewed on 31.07.2007.

111 For more details on the growth of nursing homes, see the Appendix (I–IV) attached with the unpublished Phd thesis, titled "Health Care in Crisis: The Changing Pattern of Private Health Care in Post-Independence Kolkata". Available at http://hdl.handle

.net/10603/176075. Mention may be made that this entire book is based on this Phd thesis which was awarded in the year 2011. Another work by Dr Kunal Sarkar titled *The Sickness of Health* (Kolkata: BEE Books, 2021) has some resemblance with the present work.

112 To understand the changes in the patient profile over the years, I have divided it into 'then' and 'now'. But, in case of some nursing homes and private hospitals, no remarkable change in the socio-economic profile of the patients is noticeable. In these cases, the division is not provided.

113 Though Woodlands Nursing Home was established in 1944, it was converted to Woodlands Medical Centre.

114 Though Belle Vue Clinic was established in 1967, since it is a private hospital (which was an exception in the late 1960s), the case is treated separately without following the conventional chronological order.

References

Arnold, David. *Colonizing the Body: State Medicine and Epidemic Diseases in Nineteenth Century India*. Delhi: OUP, 1993.

Bagchi, Amiya Kumar. "Studies on the Economy of West Bengal since Independence". *Economic and Political Weekly* Vol. 44, No. 47–48 (21 November 1998).

Bagchi, Amrita. *Health Care in Crisis: The Changing Pattern of Private Health Care in Post-Independence Kolkata*. Unpublished PhD thesis. http://hdl.handle.net/10603 /176075.

Bagchi, Amrita. "Public Health in Post Independence Kolkata". In *Proceedings of the Indian History Congress,* 2018 78th Session held in Jadavpur University, Kolkata, 28–30 December, 2017.

Bala, Poonam. *Imperialism and Medicine in Bengal: A Socio-Historical Perspective*. London and New Delhi: Sage Publications, 1991.

Baru, Rama V. *Factors Influencing Variations in Health Services*: *A Study of Selected Districts in Andhra Pradesh*. Unpublished M.Phil Dissertation, Jawaharlal Nehru University, 1987.

Baru, Rama V. *Private Health Care in India. Social Characteristics and Trends*. New Delhi: Sage Publications, 1998.

Bennet, Sara, Barbara McPake, and Anne Mills. *Private Health Providers: In Developing Countries-Serving the Public Interest?* London: Zed Books, 1997.

Bera, Anjan, ed. *The Nation*, 8 November 1948. Calcutta: Netaji Institute for Asian Studies, 2001.

Berger, Rachel. *Ayurveda Made Modern: Political Histories of Indigenous Medicine in North India, 1900–1955*. Cambridge Imperial and Post-colonial Studies Series. New York: Palgrave Macmillan, 2013.

Berman, Peter, and M.E. Khan. *Paying for India's Health Care*. New Delhi: Sage Publications, 1993.

Bhattacharya, Basabi. "Urbanisation and Human Development in West Bengal: A District Level Study and Comparison with Inter-State Variation". *Economic and Political Weekly* Vol. 44, No. 47–48 (21 November 1998).

Blood Test e Malaria Virus Paowa Gechhe. (Malaria Virus has been detected in the Blood Test) *Anandabazaar Patrika* (Bengali daily), 30 October 1967.

Cartwright, Ann. *Human Relations and Hospital Care*. London: Routledge and Kegan Paul Limited, 1964.

Chattopadhyay, Molly. *Occupational Socialisation: A Study of Hospital Nurses*. Calcutta: Sarat Book House, 1993.

Chaudhuri, Sukanta. *Calcutta: The Living City, The Present and Future*, Vol. II. Calcutta: Oxford University Press, 1990.

Chhetri, Mani Kumar. *Doctor*. Kolkata: Critical Care and Medical Education Trust, 2019.

Chittaranjan Seba Sadan o Jatiyakaran (Nationalization of Chittaranjan Seva Sadan). *Anandabazaar Patrika*, 22 May 1967.

Choleray 39 jon akranto (39 people *infected by cholera*). *Anandabazaar Patrika*, May 3, 1967.

Crawford, D.G. "Notes on the Early Hospitals of Calcutta". *Indian Medical Gazette* 38, no.1 (1903). 3–7.

Dasgupta, Uma, ed. *History of Science, Philosophy and Culture in Indian Civilization, xv, Science and Modern India: An Institutional History, c 1784-c 1947*. New Delhi: Center for Studies in Civilizations, 2011.

Department of Health, Government of West Bengal. *Towards Better Health in West Bengal: Progress since 1947*. Calcutta: Directorate of Health Services, State Bureau of Health Intelligence, 1962.

Drez, Jean, and Amartya Sen. *India: Development and Participation*. New Delhi: Oxford University Press, 2002.

Giri, Pabitra. "Urbanisation in West Bengal, 1951–1991". *Economic and Political Weekly* Vol. 44, No. 47–48 (21 November 1998).

Government of West Bengal, Directorate of Health Services, State Bureau of Health Intelligence, Health on the March (1967–1872).

Guha, Ratnabir. "Native Bodies, Medical Market and 'Conflicting' Medical 'Systems': Venereal Diseases and the "Vernacularisation' of Western Medical Knowledge in Colonial Bengal". *Presidency Historical Review* 1, no. 1 (2015). 11–61.

Hochmuth, Christian. "Patterns of Medical Culture in Colonial Bengal, 1835–1880". *Bulletin of the History of Medicine* 80 (2006). 39–72.

Interview with Dr Sudhir Ghosh on 31.07.2007 at Dreamland Nursing Home, Calcutta, West Bengal.

Interview with Prof Ranjit Sen at Calcutta University, Calcutta, West Bengal on 27.09.2007.

Jeffrey, Roger. *Politics of Health in India*. Berkeley: University of California Press, 1988.

Jesani, A., and S. Anantharam. *Private Sector and Privatization of the Health Care Services*. Bombay: FRCH, 1993.

Journal of Indian Medical Association (JIMA), Supplement vol. XVIII, no. 2, Editorial (Calcutta: 1948).

Kumar, Deepak, ed. *Medicine in India: A Historical Overview*. New Delhi: Tulika Books, 2001.

Malaria: Prasthan o Prabesh (Malaria: Exit and Entry). *Anadabazaar Patrika*, November 12, 1967.

Mishra, R., R. Chatterjee, and M. Rao. *India Health Report*. New Delhi: Oxford University Press, 2003.

Moir, D.M. "Notes on the Origin of the Old Presidency General Hospital Calcutta". *Bengal Past and Present* 109, Part 1–2 (1990): 208–209.

Mukharji, Projit Bihari. *Nationalizing the Body: The Medical Market, Print and Daktari Medicine*. New York: Anthem Press, 2009.

Mukharji, Projit Bihari. "Structuring Plurality: Locality, Caste, Class and Ethnicity in Nineteenth-Century Bengali Dispensaries". *Health and History* 9, no. 1 (2007). 80–105.

Mukhopadhyay, Alok, ed. *Report of the Independent Commission on Health in India*. New Delhi: Voluntary Health Associations of India, 1997.

"National Medical College-e gherao abyahata" (Gherao continues in National Medical College). *Anandabazaar Patrika*, 14 May 1967.

"National Medical College: Kartripaksher Baktabya" (National Medical College: Opinion of the Authorities). *Anandabazaar Patrika*, 7 June 1967.

"National Medicale Ordinanace Balabat" (Ordinance enforced in National Medical). *Anandabazaar Patrika*, 10 June 1967.

"National Medicalke *sarkari* niyantrane anar prastab" (Proposal to bring National Medical under government control). *Anandabazaar Patrika*, 3 May 1967.

Paria, Biswanath. *An Appeal.* Calcutta: Medical Service Centre, 1985.

Pati, Biswamaoy, and Mark Harrison. *Health Medicine and Empire Perspectives on Colonial Medicine.* New Delhi: OUP, 2001.

Phadke, Anant. *Private Medical Sector in India.* Bombay: FRCH, 1994.

Porter, Roy. *Health for Sale: Quackery in England, 1660–85.* Manchester: Manchester University Press, 1989.

Prasad, Purendra, and Jessani Amar, eds. *Equity and Access: Health Care Studies in India.* New Delhi: OUP, 2018.

Presidential Address by Dr A.C. Ukil, published in *Journal of Indian Medical Association* 26, no. 5 (March 1956).

Presidential Address by Dr A.K. Bose at the 13th Bengal Provincial Medical Conference held in Midnapore on 7 and 8 November 1953, in *Journal of Indian Medical Association (JIMA)* xxiii, no. 5 (February 1954).

Presidential Address by Dr B.P. Trivedi at the XVII Bengal Provincial Medical Conference, Bishnupur, 1958, published in *Journal of Indian Medical Association* (Supplement), 3, no. 7 (October 1958).

Qadeer, Imrana. "Health Services System in India: An Expression of Socio-Economic Inequalities". *Social Action* 35 (July-September 1985).

"Rajya sab pareni, tai prayojan besarkari haspataler" (The state *has failed, so private hospitals are needed*). *Anandabazar Patrika*, 20 January 1989.

Rao, Mohan. "The State of Health in India". *South Asian Journal: Indo-Pak Dialogue*, October–December 2006.

Ray, Kabita. *History of Public Health: Colonial Bengal 1921–1947.* Calcutta: K.P.Bagchi and Sons, 1998.

Samanta, Arabinda. *Malarial Fever in Colonial Bengal 1820–1939: Social History of An Epidemic.* Kolkata: FIRMA KLM, 2002.

Sarkar, Kunal. *The Sickness of Health.* Kolkata: BEE Books, 2021.

"Sarkari Parichalanay National Medical o Chittaranjan Hospital" (National Medical and Chittaranjan Hospital under Government Management). *Anandabazaar Patrika*, 23 May 1967.

Sen, Gaur. "Sahar Kolkatar Katha". *Swasthya Dwipika*, no. 12, Agrahayan–Paush 1374 (December 1967).

Sharma, Madhuri. *Indigenous and Western Medicine in Colonial India, Culture and Environment in South Asia.* New Delhi: Foundation Books, 2012.

4 Causes behind the Changing Profile of Private Healthcare Sectors

Introduction

Most hospitals in India were either run by government or private charities and trusts until the 1970s. In the early 1980s, the state encouraged private nursing homes and small and medium hospitals to supplement government healthcare (mentioned as *incremental privatization* in Chapter 1) and facilities to meet the growing needs of the sick and poor. But soon a significant shift in government policy led to the recognition of hospital as an industry. In 1991 or in the post-liberalization era, there was a drastic cut in the central government budgetary allocation for healthcare, which favoured the establishment of private hospitals in India. The liberalization policy and health sector reforms provided opportunities in the healthcare markets for local and international corporations. State facilitated the growth of the corporate health sector to establish tertiary-level super speciality hospitals to achieve 'high quality' care and this continued through the 1990s and 2000s. The government opened up in 2000 the foreign direct investment (FDI) route in hospitals and mobilization of capital, stimulating the growth of corporate hospitals (mentioned as *programmed privatization* in Chapter 1). The Insurance Regulatory Development Authority allowed third party administrators and customized medical insurance in the last decades, supposedly to provide greater access to the poor and social protection. What is common across these sets of reforms is the gradual de-emphasis on public healthcare institutions and the promotion of private and corporate hospitals by effectively allocating government resources.[1]

In the previous chapter an attempt was made to locate the conditions of the public health and healthcare services in a newly independent metropolis. Parallelly, the causes behind the 'rise and fall' of the small, private nursing homes in the pre-liberalization era in Calcutta were also depicted. This chapter intends to look into the factors or causes behind the corporatization of the private healthcare sector in the city and its transformation into a lucrative industry. The retreat of the welfare state and its consequent impact on the healthcare sector, focusing on the degeneration of public healthcare in West Bengal will be addressed in Section I and Section II, respectively. In Section III, the failure of the public health sector will be studied in the broader framework of the neoliberal turn that infused corporate

DOI: 10.4324/9781003169475-5

capital in healthcare and how the Structural Adjustment Programmes (SAP) prepared the ground for the fast growth of corporate healthcare.

Section I

Retreating State

The entire public healthcare infrastructure in India has shown signs of unsatisfactory performance and degeneration from the time of its inception. The welfare state had deprived this sector by allocating funds incommensurate with the demand of the population. On the other hand, due to these inadequacies the private health sector emerged as an obvious alternative to meet the healthcare needs of the population at large. The politics of the government to destabilize the importance of the public healthcare sector in the post-Independence period was one of the significant causes behind the rapid emergence of the private healthcare sector.

In India, at the time of Independence there was a significant presence of the private sector, which was dominated by individual practitioners. As per the estimates of the Bhore Committee, the proportion of allopathic doctors in private practice was 73 per cent and the remaining 27 per cent were in government service.

For decades, the government has systematically nurtured the private health sector. This unwritten policy of the government runs parallel to the neglect and gradual withdrawal of the state from the responsibility of people's health. Such consistent support and encouragement to the private health sector are important reasons for the failure to provide universal basic healthcare to all people of the country.[2]

The information on the nature and extent of growth is limited but a few studies have demonstrated the significant presence of the private sector in some parts of the country.[3] Even at the national level, if one compares the rate of growth of government and private hospitals from the mid-1970s, the latter seems to have grown at a faster pace.[4] India probably has the largest private healthcare segment in the world.[5] However, it is interesting to note that though this sector is large and an important constituent of the country's healthcare delivery system, the data on the share of the private sector in the overall healthcare is highly unsatisfactory and highly unreliable. Data on the sectoral distribution of doctors is not easily available, as many states do not file the required information to the Ministry of Health[6]. As the Tenth Plan document notes, there is no uniform nationwide system of registering either practitioners or institutions in the private sector. Nor is there any system for obtaining and analyzing information about this large sector.

It is clear from Table 4.1 that the private and voluntary healthcare sectors have successfully multiplied their numbers both in terms of organizations and bed strength over the ten years from 1973 to 1983. In some states like Andhra Pradesh, Maharashtra, Tamil Nadu, Uttar Pradesh and West Bengal there has been a substantial presence of these sectors, and their numbers in two respective years have increased significantly. In Andhra Pradesh the number of private and voluntary hospitals has increased from 113 to 266 and bed strength from 9,213 to 11,103. In

Table 4.1 Growth of Private and Voluntary Hospitals and Beds in Major States

Sl No.	State	1973		1983	
1	Andhra Pradesh	113	9,213	266	11,103
2	Bihar	N.A.	N.A.	125	8,447
3	Gujarat	41	1,219	669	16,929
4	Haryana	17	1,877	18	2,566
5	Karnataka	38	5,106	53	6,894
6	Kerala	N.A.	N.A.	606	18,203
7	Madhya Pradesh	8	1,601	N.A.	N.A.
8	Maharashtra	68	8,300	682	32,033
9	Orissa	35	1,741	34	1,227
10	Punjab	20	2,070	35	2,913
11	Tamil Nadu	69	9,618	61	8,562
12	Uttar Pradesh	151	19,897	160	12,083
13	West Bengal	78	8,452	126	6,424
14	All-India	718	66,926	3,022	1,34,266

Source: Health Information of India (various years).[7]

Table 4.2 Distribution of Hospitals and Hospital Beds according to Ownership

Ownership	1983				1987			
	Hospitals	%	Beds	%	Hospitals	%	Beds	%
Government	3,632	49	348,861	68	3,664	38	367,380	64
Local	433	6	25,894	5	516	5	27,682	5
Voluntary	569	8	53,513	11	935	10	74,498	13
Private	2,764	37	84,206	16	4,488	47	104,018	18
Total	7,398	100	512,474	100	9,603	100	573,578	100

Source: Directory of Hospitals in India, 1985 and 1988.[8]

Maharashtra there has been a jump in the number of hospitals from 68 to 682 and the number of beds rose from 8,300 to 32,033. Uttar Pradesh has also exhibited a rise in the number of hospitals from 151 to 160, but in this state, there has been a decrease in the number of beds from 19,897 to 12,083. However, Tamil Nadu has experienced a decline both in the number of hospitals and beds. Although there has been an increase in the number of hospitals from 78 to 126 in West Bengal, bed strength declined from 8,452 to 6,424.

However, the private healthcare services had exhibited a steady growth from the mid-1970s and the mushrooming of smaller nursing homes all over the country further complicated the relationship between private and public healthcare sectors. Comparing the growth of the public and private hospitals in India, it is easy to infer that the latter had multiplied at a faster pace. It can be seen from Table 4.2 that the number of government hospitals and beds in 1983 was 3,932 (49 per cent) and 348,861 (68 per cent), respectively. But the percentage of hospitals and hospital beds reduced to 38 and 64, respectively, in 1987. On the other hand, the hospitals and hospital beds in the private sector increased substantially between 1983 and 1987 from 2,764 (37 per cent) hospitals and 84,206 (16 per cent) hospital beds to 4,488 (47 per cent) and 104,018 (18 per cent), respectively. Other sectors – voluntary and local – also expanded over time.

Studies have shown that a fairly large percentage of doctors employed in the public sector practise privately. They often use government hospitals to treat their patients.[9] A majority of the doctors who practise privately, do so along with their government jobs. According to them a government job offers security, contacts and status and also helps in gaining good experience.[10]

There was no effort by the government to curb the growth of the private sector. The proportion of private nursing homes and hospitals was insignificant at the time of Independence. However, these institutions started growing during the 1970s and were restricted to urban areas and states where there was capitalist growth in agriculture. The cutback in public spending coupled with government subsidies has resulted in the growth of the private sector at secondary and tertiary levels of care. In India, it is mainly an urban phenomenon but, in some states, there has been a growth in services in peri-urban and even rural areas.[11]

From 1945 through the 1960s, there was considerable growth in welfare services with an emphasis on food security, maternal and child health services and an expansion of health services at the primary, secondary and tertiary levels of care. Public investments were made in both service provisioning and training of human resources.

Actions in health and other fields in the first two decades of Independence placed the country very high among the newly sovereign countries. The motive force generated by the leadership commitment and the experience gained by the health administrators from their work in the Indian Medical Service (IMS) enabled them to give a concrete shape to the political vision of the rulers. This led to some far-reaching developments in health services. This period was termed the Golden Two Decades of Public Health in India. Some of the landmarks requiring mention were: vertical programmes, primary health centres, social orientation of medical education, indigenous systems of medicine, Family Planning/Welfare Programme, water supply and sanitation, nutrition, Minimum Needs Programme, the Multi-Purpose Workers Scheme, the Community Health Volunteers Scheme and the Statement of National Health Policy.[12]

The political vision to establish a comprehensive health service system in the aftermath of Independence was unfortunately short-lived. Over the next three decades, there was a sharp decline in the quality of health services in the country. One of the major forces contributing to this decline was the obsessive preoccupation with the Family Planning Programme at the cost of serious neglect of the health service needs of the people, particularly the poor. The medical schools contributed significantly to the growth of the private sector since on an average 80 per cent of the medical graduates entered private practice or migrated abroad.

Since the mid-1970s, the state provided various incentives like concessional land, tax-breaks and duty exemptions for imports for setting up of private hospitals. The private pharmaceutical industry also received substantial state patronage for its growth through process patent laws, subsidized bulk drugs from public sector companies and protection from MNCs.[13]

During the 1980s, public health spending peaked and this was reflected in major health infrastructure expansion in rural India via the Minimum Needs Programme. In fact, the entitlements mentioned above were achieved during this decade in most states. However, in the 1990s, the public health sector was woefully neglected with new public investments being virtually stopped and expenditures declining.[14]

The expenditure on health as a percentage of total government expenditure was 5.5 in 1977; it declined to 3.2 in 1981, rose to 5.5 and peaked at 6.5 in 1989. During the 1990s, it declined from 5 per cent to 4.1 per cent.[15] The government health spending on medical care and public health, as a proportion to the total government expenditure, declined in real terms from 3.2 per cent to 2.7 per cent. Worse, the reduced spending had a higher proportion of salaries that increased from 39.93 per cent to 58.97 per cent and a corresponding decline in capital expenditures from 4.37 per cent to 2.58 per cent. In terms of GDP, public spending increased from 0.98 per cent in 1975 to 1.36 per cent in 1986, only to fall to 1.28 per cent by 1991 – this contracted even further to 0.09 per cent by 2000, resulting in the marginalization of the state as the primary player in the health service.[16] This poor investment pattern in healthcare retarded the expansion of public health services, and this was the phase when 'welfare state'-driven growth of the private health sector started flourishing (see Figure 4.1).

In this context the changing role of the welfare state should be pointed out. The decline of public health and subsequent healthcare (contributing to the growth of the private health sector) is closely linked with the 'retreat of the welfare state'.

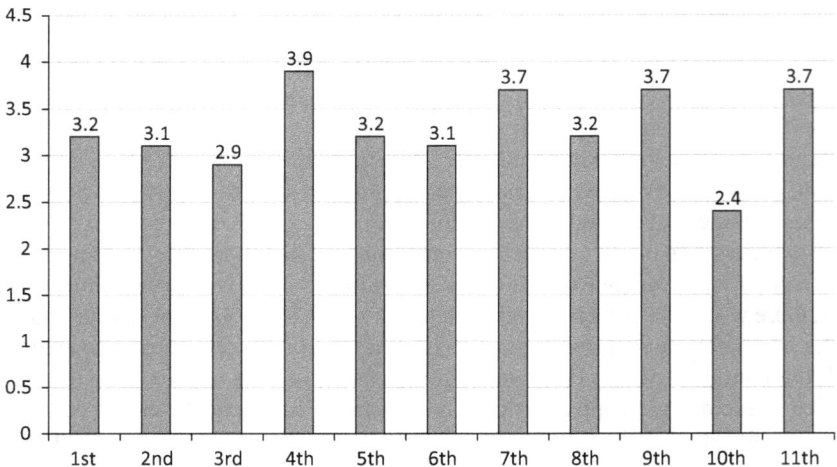

Figure 4.1 Showing the proportion of investment in the health sector to the total budget investment/outlay through various five-year plans in India Hooda, "Health System in Transition in India", 509–10.

The health status of the population in developing countries is well below that in the industrialized countries and the distribution, as well as the quality of health-care in developing countries, leaves much to be desired. It is well known that the scarcity of resources for healthcare in developing countries is a primary cause of this state of affairs.[17]

The cutting back of public expenditure and selective state intervention made the greater role of the market obvious in curative healthcare. Until the late 1970s, a nationalized system for providing welfare services arose across both developed and developing countries.[18] Developing countries in Africa, Asia and Latin America managed to build national health service systems with their meagre resources. With the oil shock of the late 1970s, both developed and developing countries started to feel the fiscal crunch, and in many countries a cutback in welfare spending was seen as a measure to deal with the situation. As a result, most developing countries had to cut back even their minimal spending on welfare and this had an adverse impact on the growth of service.[19]

Moreover, it is also necessary to review briefly the public healthcare fundamentals as primary healthcare is the fulcrum around which our entire healthcare delivery system is organized. According to the Rural Health Statistics Bulletin (2017–2018)[20] there were 1.39 health centres (either of sub-centres (SCs) and primary health centres (PHCs)) per 10,000 people nationally with a shortage of 32,900 sub-centres and 6,430 PHCs. Besides the existing 46 per cent of shortfall of doctors in PHCs, 74 per cent of the current graduate doctors reside in urban India leaving a large chunk of the rural population underserved. The vacancy rate of doctors is 24.9 per cent across rural PHCs.

India's ability to expand universal access to primary healthcare is seriously hampered by the persistent gaps in infrastructure required to deliver a basket of services. There is still a normative gap of 3,469 community health centres (CHCs) for a population of 0.1 million, 5,887 PHCs for every 30,000 people and 27,430 sub-centres for every 5,000 people. Seventy per cent of the gap is in the poorly performing states that also have the disease burden. Besides, the existing facilities are not equipped and have inadequate infrastructure with 10 per cent of the PHCs and 35 per cent of the sub-centres housed in thatched huts located more than 3 kilometres away from the village, seriously impacting access.[21]

Studies on the private sector in several developing countries show that the world recession of the late 1970s hindered the financing of public services and resulted in the growth of markets in the welfare sector.[22]

This is evident from the fact that in 1973 the percentage of beds in public hospitals was 71.2 while that in private hospitals was 28.8. In 1993, the percentage of beds in public hospitals got reduced to 42.3 and that in the private hospitals increased to 57.7. In the next phase, the private health sector, including the hospital sector, expanded rapidly on the one hand, and on the other the public health system was being reformed to fit the market model through the introduction of user charges and contracting out of services. The figure changed in 1996, when the percentage of hospital beds in the public sector decreased to 39 and that in the private sector increased to 61.[23] By 2010–2011, the share of allopathic facilities was around 76 per cent, consisting of hospitals (7.8 per cent), medical (55.6 per cent), dental (4.1 per cent), nursing (4.1 per cent) and diagnostic (4.4 per cent) labs/centres, whereas the shares of service providers of homoeopathy and Ayurveda medicines were recorded to be around 11.2 per cent and 7.4 per cent, respectively. It is interesting to note that after Independence, roughly 1,352 private health enterprises were recorded in 1950, which cumulatively increased to 10.4 lakh in 2010–2011.[24] Approximately, an estimated 54.3 per cent of the medical institutions, 75 per cent of the hospitals, 51 per cent of the hospital beds, 75 per cent of the dispensaries and 80 per cent of all qualified doctors are in the private sector.[25] The share of government health enterprises in 2016 was found to be only 20 per cent.[26]

Section II

Weak Public Health Facilities in West Bengal vis-a-vis Kolkata in the Late 1990s to 2000s

There have always been substantial gaps in the proportion of public healthcare infrastructure and the effective demand for its utilization in Kolkata. In 2005–2006, in Kolkata there were nine medical colleges having 7,948 beds. Of these, 1,158 beds were distributed in five state general hospitals of the city. There were 15 other hospitals (mental, ID, dental, TB, leprosy, etc.) with a total of 2,878 beds. Hospitals under nine state government departments (jail, police and ESI) other than health had 1,711 beds. The number of hospitals under local bodies are eight, having 354 beds in all. Hospitals under the central government are five in number and have 1,164 beds. There were 288 hospitals under the NGO/private sector having 8,213 beds. Thus, the total number of hospitals in Kolkata was 335 and the total number of beds in both public and private sectors was 23,426. Although the share of beds in the public sector was larger than that in the private sector, the number of institutions in the private health sector was more compared to the public sector, which numbered only 47 (see Table 4.3).

It is noteworthy that from 2006 onwards, *Health on the March* published figures on another category, the NGO/private sector, where the 'private sector'

Table 4.3 Medical Institutions and the Number of Sanctioned Beds in Kolkata (2005–2006)[27]

Medical College and Hospital		State General Hospitals		Other Hospitals[a]		Hospitals under Other Departments of State Government[b]		Local Body		Government of India		NGO/Private	
No.	Total No. of Beds	No.	Total No. of Beds	No.	Total No. of Beds	No.	Total No. of Beds	No.	Total No. of Beds	No.	Total No of Beds	No	Total No. of Beds
05	7948	05	1,158	15	2878	09	1,711	08	354	05	1,164	288	8,213

[a] This includes six teaching hospitals and five decentralized hospitals.
[b] Includes government undertaking organization.

indicates the profit-making healthcare services (nursing homes and private hospitals). Earlier, this category was identified as the voluntary sector, which signified the private-aided or non-profit sector.

Although there have been some obvious developments in recent years, the ratio of population served per bed does not exhibit a positive situation. From the table below we can see the changes noticeable in the pattern of developments in private and public healthcare institutions in the district of Kolkata from 2005 to 2018 (see Table 4.4).

Mention should be made that in the case of Kolkata only there are no district, sub-divisional, rural hospitals and block primary health centre and primary health centres. It is interesting to point out that there were five state general hospitals with a total bed strength of 1,158 in Kolkata as recorded in *Health on the March* (2005–2006). But there is no corresponding data from Kolkata in *Health on the March* in 2018. From the two tables (4.3 and 4.4) it can be inferred that the private healthcare organizations have increased up to 39 per cent in 2018 as compared to 2005. The total number of medical institutions in 2005 was 335 and that in 2018 was 449. Out of which there were only 49 public healthcare institutions in 2018 and the rest 400 were private. There was just 4.25 per cent of increase in the growth of public health organizations from 2005 to 2018 as compared to a 39 per cent of rise in the private healthcare sector. Thus it is clear that the state-funded healthcare sector is exhibiting a sharp decline in recent years. The number of beds in the public sector increased only by 18 per cent from 2005 to 2018 while in the private health sector there was an increase of more than 104 per cent.

Even in the case of rural healthcare there was a substantial stagnation in the case of the growth of sub-centres as is evident from Tables 4.5 and 4.6. The number of Block Primary Centres has been reduced to 75 (a few have been upgraded) in 2018 from 241 in 2005. The number of beds also reduced to 1,470 from 4,699 during the same period. Only the number of rural hospitals increased substantially from 93 in 2005 to 273 in 2018 and the bed strength from 3,418 in 2005 to 9,546 in 2018. Mention should be made that government has subsequently increased the number of medical colleges in West Bengal from 9 in 2005–2006 to 13 in 2011–2012 and finally 18 in 2018.[29] Parallelly, the bed strength in medical colleges also increased from 11,130 in 2005 to 12,614 in 2011–2012 and finally 17,803 in 2018. But this increase does not improve the healthcare infrastructure, rather it aggravates the inequity as the primary and secondary level are not expanded proportionately.

Table 4.4 Medical Institutions and the Number of Sanctioned Beds in Kolkata as on 31 March 2018[28]

Medical College and Hospital		Other Hospitals		Hospitals under Other Department of State Government	Local Body		Government of India		NGO/Private	
No.	Total No. of Beds	No.	Total No. of Beds	No.	Total No. of Beds	No.	Total No. of Beds	No.	Total No. of Beds	No.	Total No. of Beds
05	8,129	21	4,821	09	1,711	06	308	08	3,072	400	16,757

Table 4.5 Medical Institutions in West Bengal as on 2005–2006[30]

Hospitals/Health Centres under Department of Health and Family Welfare		Total No. of beds (Sanctioned)
Medical College Hospital	9	11,130
District Hospital	15	6,766
Sub-Divisional Hospital	45	8,506
State General Hospital	34	4,212
Other Hospitals	32	7,223
Rural Hospitals	93	3,418
Block Primary Health Centre	241	4,699
Primary Health Centre	922	5,247
Sub-Centres	10,356	0
Hospitals under Other Departments of State Government	67	6,042
Hospitals under Local Body	30	940
Hospitals under Government of India	57	6,208
Hospitals under NGO/Private	1,726	27,543
Total	**13,627**	**91,934**

As has been discussed in Chapter 3, public healthcare in Kolkata was always in a decaying state. In a study[32] published in 2012 it was depicted that the state of West Bengal where about three-quarters of the population live in villages, the remaining quarter live in urban areas and more than half reside in greater Kolkata was at the crossroads in the field of the healthcare delivery system. It is needless to say that the state economy rests on the health, ability and wellbeing of the people. West Bengal is one of the most fiscally stressed states of all the Indian states. The government health system in West Bengal has been on the verge of collapse vis-a-vis the booming of private hospitals, nursing homes, clinics, diagnostic centres, insurance companies, Third Party Administrators, touts, etc. The government even waived tax from money- and profit-making organizations in the name of 'research'. The government has not been able to thwart the unethical and corrupt activities of some private institutions like excessive and false billing, unnecessary investigations, negligence in patient care and irrational use of a ventilator, ICU, etc.[33]

The study quoted the District Development Report for West Bengal, which indicated that Malda, Uttar Dinajpur, Dakshin Dinajpur, Murshidabad, Purulia and Cooch Behar had the highest levels of health service deprivation – children not fully immunized and non-institutional deliveries.

> This reflects the inadequacies of outreach of health services provided by the state, alongside poor-quality delivery services. Children born in the poorest districts are less likely to survive than to children born in other districts; similarly, in these districts pregnant mothers are less likely to receive antenatal care and institutional support for deliveries, thereby making them more vulnerable.[34]

Table 4.6 Type-Wise Number of Medical Institutions and Beds in West Bengal[31]

Type of Medical Institution	As on 31 December 2016		As on 31 December 2017		As on 31 December 2018	
	No.	Total No. of Beds (Sanctioned)	No.	Total No. of Beds (Sanctioned)	No.	Total No. of Beds (Sanctioned)
Hospitals/Health Centres under Department of Health and Family Welfare						
Medical College Hospital	13	15,190	13	15,708	18	17,803
Other Teaching Hospitals	6	2,366	6	2,366	6	2,366
District Hospital	22	10,100	23	10,621	18	8,526
Multi/Super Speciality Hospitals	42	13,800	42	13,800	42	13,800
Sub-Divisional Hospital	37	8,210	36	7,840	36	7,840
State General Hospital	24	2,778	24	2,778	24	2,778
Other Hospitals (Leprosy, Mental, Dental, etc.)*	34	7,232	34	7,232	34	7,232
SNCU (Established at Different Hospitals)	70	2,523	70	2,523	70	2,523
SNSU (Established at Different Hospitals)	307	680	307	680	307	680
CCU (Established at Different Hospitals)	37	572	37	572	37	572
HDU (Established at Different Hospitals)	21	126	21	126	21	126
PICU (at 12 MCH and Teaching Hospitals)	–	208	–	208	–	208
MCH Hubs (at Nine Hospitals including MCH and	–	2,250	–	2,250	–	2,250
Rural Hospitals	273	9,361	273	9,446	273	9,546
Block Primary Health Centre	75	1,195	75	1,470	75	1,470
Primary Health Centre	913	7,002	913	7,191	913	7,191
Sub-Centres	10,369	–	10,369	–	10,369	–
Total Beds		83,593		84,811		84,911
Total Beds in Govt. Hospitals	72	6,212			67	5,672
Hospitals under Other Departments of State	47	1,521			30	1,083
Hospitals under Local Body	58	7,126			57	8,146
Hospitals under Government of India**5	2,058	46,346			2,139	53,992
Hospitals under NGO/Private5	72					
Total Beds		144,798				153,804

In another study[35] around the same time it was pointed out that due to high population pressure in West Bengal, the infrastructural facility was found to be insufficient as there was only one Community Health Centre for almost every three lakh population, which is supposed to be one for every lakh as per the national norm; primary health centres and sub-centres were also observed to be having a similar kind of a situation, dealing with double or triple number of population than they were capable of handling. This reduced their efficiency and thereby caused poor health service. The situation was found to be better in hilly areas due to low population density as in Darjeeling and was found to be worse in urban and suburban plain areas as in North 24-Parganas. However, for almost all the districts in West Bengal, there is at least one sub-centre for every 10,000 population, indicating that at least one step towards a proper rural health infrastructure has been taken at the grassroots level. But in the secondary level of the healthcare system, district hospitals as well as the medical college hospitals are found to be overcrowded with patient pressure indicating poor service from the primary or rural health institutions, viz. CHC/PHC/SC. A huge number of patients are being referred to the medical colleges as well as district hospitals due to lack of infrastructural support in the rural health centres and this is making the hospitals crowded, unhealthy and less efficient. In many medical college hospitals two or three patients share a bed and some even lie on the floor to get treatment. This may be the possible reason why people even with marginally higher financial strength prefer to go to private hospitals. Economically richer districts are found to be having a greater number of private medical institutions as there is a strong association between wealth of the people and preference to private healthcare. For example, Kolkata has the highest number of private medical institutions followed by Bardhaman, North 24-Parganas and Hooghly. However, these hospitals are beyond the reach of poor people. Hence, still a very small percentage of the total population is capable of visiting private hospitals.[36]

The present researcher also has conducted a survey among patients at Calcutta Medical College and Hospital. In spite of these negativities of the public hospitals and their depiction in several government documents, responses from 27 patients in the government hospital reveal a different picture. The socio-economic profiles of the patients show that they are mostly from the economically challenged section. Out of 27 cases I can mention a few to convey their experiences. Sanjib Biswas (29), a vegetable seller from Nadia, admitted in general medicine had no complaints about the services of the hospital and the staff. Narayan Debnath above 40 from Burdwan said that all the staff members, even the sweepers, attended at the time of emergency and most of the time ward boys were available to change saline. Avik Das, a 16-year-old boy (whose father works in a private firm) from Hooghly, admitted to the general medicine department for haemophilia, also had the same experience. His mother felt at home in the hospital, and they were especially obliged to the nurses and doctors of the hospital. Paresh Das (49), who works in an iron factory in Howrah, had no complaints about the services. His previous experiences in this hospital were equally good. Suren Sau, who had retired from the Bengal Chemical factory, felt that the services in public hospitals were still unparalleled. These patients and many others with whom I have talked at the Medical College generally come from the lower-income group and sometimes from below the poverty line. Their experiences do not match with the reality of the existing notion of the public healthcare services because the condition in their rural background is more pathetic than the services in the Medical College. Secondly the perception of the quality of medical services is also relative. Since they never had the opportunity to avail of treatment in a private sector hospital, it is also difficult for them to identify the differences in the quality of services. Thirdly, most of these patients who have their monthly income below Rs 2,000 do not have the aspiration for better services, because the services in the rural hospital are even worse and to them this is the standard treatment they could get within their affordability. So, these patients from their own socio-economic and cultural position judge the systems as flawless and adequate since this service is capable of fulfilling the needs of this section. Getting a free bed, a blanket, regular meals in the hospital, medicine and care do really satisfy their need.

The National Sample Survey (NSS) 60th Round, conducted in 2004–2005, found that the 'reasons for non-utilisation of government facilities for outpatient care' in West Bengal were bad treatment (as perceived by the patients), poor accessibility and long waiting time. The situation has not changed much in so many years. Furthermore, a significant portion of the population in rural West Bengal depends on unqualified medical practitioners.[37]

In the case of Kolkata, the situation of public hospitals was far from satisfactory. This has been mentioned in a study of socio-economic profiles of patients in R.G. Kar and AMRI hospitals.[38] The high concentration of patients from districts in R.G. Kar is due to the collapse of the referral system. The District Human Development Reports for Malda and Birbhum showed a 'top heavy' healthcare system with significant differences in the bed turnover rates in block primary health centres (BPHCs) and at district and sub-divisional hospitals. Our study also finds a large proportion of patients utilizing the developed transport links between North 24-Parganas and Kolkata to access health facilities in R.G. Kar.[39]

As a result, instead of being a referral institution, R.G. Kar has become a centre for diagnosis.[40]

It is relevant to mention in this context that the Pratichi Health Report has also taken account of the non-functioning primary health centres in the districts of Birbhum and Dumka (Jharkhand).[41]

The poor condition of the public healthcare sector was addressed in the Report of the Standing Committee on Health and Family Welfare, 1999–2000.[42] The Committee observed that the coordination between the different groups of health personnel was utterly deficient. There was a lack of understanding and cooperation between different sections of Group D, Group C and nursing staff, medical personnel and administrative officers. In many cases there were hostility and indifferent attitude amongst them.

The problems with the drainage system in the hospitals are acute, and the disposal of hospital waste is defective. There are defects in the construction of the buildings and other civil work. These problems are multiplied due to the apathy and negligent attitude of the incumbents and the recipients as well. Deficiency in the attitude to keep the institution clean is the real problem.[43]

The public health system in West Bengal bears an exceptionally large burden, because in addition to the high demographic pressure on the state, which has already been noted, the bulk of curative services are in public hands. The very large responsibility and coverage of the public health system in the state are evident from the fact that 76 per cent of the health institutions in West Bengal are run by the government. Obviously, the total physical infrastructure available for healthcare in the state is still inadequate relative to requirements and it has already been noted that there are also problems with the quality of the health service delivery in several key areas.[44]

The problems of the government hospitals as far as the delivery of services is concerned have been elaborated in the study 'A Survey of a Public Hospital in Kolkata'.[45] This empirical study elaborates on the difficulties and the problems which patients and the patient parties face in any government hospital.

Curtailment of life-saving drugs, stoppage of permanent recruitment, shortage of paramedical staff, freezing posts along with rampant corruption and nepotism and favouring contractual jobs brought about the decay in the services of the government hospitals.[46]

One of the senior physicians of Kolkata has pointed out that the government hospital network is vast in absolute terms but pitifully small in comparison to the urgent needs of the people. So private hospitals and nursing homes also have a large and ever-increasing role.[47] It has been pointed out further that the rural hospitals lack medicine and supportive services. As a result, critically ill poor people have to undertake a hazardous, costly and time-taking journey to the few city-based hospitals. The pressure on the hospitals is so great that the system is at the point of collapse. Overworked junior doctors or nurses can hardly give the patients the minimum attention they need. This is coupled with indiscipline, corruption and callousness on the part of a section of the employees. Matters are made even worse by red-tapism and bureaucratic inefficiency. The inevitable result is public frustration, aggression and even violence.

West Bengal's healthcare system has taken centre stage in recent days. While opinions may differ on the state of healthcare, especially after recent incidents of alleged negligence and misbehaviour by hospital staff as well as relatives of patients, there is some amount of unanimity on the need for a mindset change.

Relatives of patients have often complained of unsympathetic behaviour by the hospital staff, including doctors and nurses. There have been instances of doctors or other medical staff being beaten up. On the other hand, there have been cases where house staff and medical students have attacked not only patients' relatives but also media persons. So there is agreement on one point: the healthcare system needs to be revamped, and relatives of patients, as well as medical staff, need to change their mindset.[48]

During the previous Left Front regime, not only Opposition parties but even partners of the ruling Front were sometimes critical of the poor state of healthcare.[49] Former chief minister Buddhadeb Bhattacharjee, during his tenure, had admitted in public that healthcare was a problem area in the state. But, he said, it was not as bad as was being made out to be. There was some consolation for him. The secretary, the Union Health and Family Welfare Ministry, J.V.R. Prasad Rao, at a seminar on health organized by the Bengal Chamber of Commerce and Industry said that 'the state of affairs is the same across the country'.[50]

The then ruling Left Front partners had also expressed their worries about the state of affairs. The doctors' cell of the Communist Party of India felt that government hospitals were overcrowded and facilities had not improved much over the years to cope with the growing number of patients. Unless district and rural hospitals became capable of handling patients, the rush to Kolkata would continue. Hence, physical infrastructure in hospitals, both in Kolkata and in the districts, needed to be improved considerably, it said. Moreover, doctors and nurses needed to be more sympathetic to patients despite the fact that they had to work under tremendous pressure.[51] The lacunae in the public healthcare sector are partly responsible for incremental privatization. Kolkata had already experienced the emergence of small nursing homes and private hospitals from the late 1970s and they acted as trendsetters for the further development of the private health sector. However, in the pre-liberalization era, this sector had not adopted the character of an industry. The public healthcare services, which were weak and inadequate from the time of Independence due to poor funding collapsed with the fiscal cutbacks of the welfare state. Pre-liberalization India had a substantial presence in the private healthcare sector, which provided the conducive atmosphere for transforming healthcare into a lucrative commodity in the following decades under the forces of globalization. The corporatization of the healthcare services, intrusion of market forces and the planned privatization programme are products of the 'neoliberal' phase of healthcare development. Shrinking of the public healthcare sector was further aggravated in the post-liberalization phase preparing the ground for the corporate health sector to flourish unabashedly.

This first phase of reforms based on receding state control did not mean retreat of the state (as is often argued) but fostered a much more hardened state, re-engineered as the safety net for capitalism and nicknamed the 'steward'![52] Its direction became anti-poor, anti-welfare and least concerned about the wellbeing of the people. This transformed state, through consistent policy changes, consolidated the markets and the interests of those who had access to it. It is therefore heavily guided by class interests.[53]

Section III

Neoliberal Shift

Systematic failures in India's health infrastructure and the retreating nature of the welfare state were further accelerated due to the shift towards a neoliberal economy in the late 1980s. Neocolonialism in thought and practice, with the World Bank and other bilateral and multilateral agencies donating a particular source of ideological and financial support, has encouraged those who have pushed for liberalization of the Indian economy. These neoliberal policies have transformed India's healthcare system.[54] These policies found their echo in the attitude of the political class and large sections of bureaucracy whose trust in the public sector was eroding. Both the Congress governments of Indira Gandhi and Rajiv Gandhi played a significant role in affecting several policy changes for hospitals to be recognized as an industry, facilitated access to finances, offered concessions for infrastructure and slashed import duties on high-technology equipment. Large government investments made in medical education allowed the private sector to access subsidized, cheap but good quality doctors. Freeze in government recruitments left little choice to the medical graduates but to join the private sector or fly abroad. Public–private partnerships (PPPs) were expanded to channelize government revenues to provide further impetus to private sector growth. These public subsidies were meant to boost FDI and attract professionals back to India. The liberalization of the health sector is reflected in the Health Policy 1982, which actively sought to engage both the for-profit and non-profit sectors.[55]

Moreover, a crisis in global capitalism has required a shift to 'surplus extraction without welfare'. The privatization of healthcare since the late 1980s must be seen in this wider context of structural changes in capitalism. Welfare sector expansion played an important role in the rejuvenating economy. The emergence of institutions like the IMF, World Bank and General Agreement on Tariffs and Trade (GATT) no doubt helped concentrate power in the hands of the western block over the 1930s to 1960s, where most of the transnational corporations were located. The search for new markets created inter-imperialist conflicts within capitalist economies. The hegemony of the US control over this search was threatened, and the oil crisis added to the woes of the western countries, which intensified the business of loans and aid and fresh wars in West Asia.[56]

The Asian countries, despite their relative economic resilience, started getting trapped in the debt burden. Information technology became the instrument of this growing phenomenon of finance capital. The North, especially the US, protected its own agriculture and labour to the extent possible and attempted to practise austerity, the ex-socialist states were forced to face the consequences of the economic shock and the developing periphery of the capitalist system was offered Structural Adjustment programmes (SAP). The strategy was to deepen the links between public and private sectors, shift state subsidies to the private sector, focus on technology-based services (with the promotion of high-tech) and commoditize them and create low-cost alternatives for the poor to contain social unrest. Thus, balancing corporate interests, elite demands for personalized high-tech services and needs of the majority were attempted.[57]

The nature of technological inventions in sectors such as medicine (antibiotics, vaccines, chemicals for vector control, nutritional supplements), drinking water supply (filtration plants and piped water supply) and sanitation (sanitary pits and waste disposal technologies) and transport (roads, railways, bus systems) made extensive population coverage possible and economically feasible, thereby scaling up these services. The second crisis of the 1970s preceded by the electronic-based communication revolution was tackled partially by this very technology for faster movement of financial capital across the globe.[58] It increased wealth without actually increasing production. The invention of the chip revolutionized the invasive power of medical technology and made it more individualized, costly and restrictive of employment within the sector.[59]

India's official acceptance of SAP not only further integrated the country into the periphery of the capitalist system but also set the stage for a major transformation of its welfare sector including the health sector challenging to expand and transform the scope of the medical market.[60]

In line with the neoliberal priority of opening up investment opportunities for the private sector, India threw open the health insurance sector to private players in 1999, setting the foreign direct investment (FDI) cap in health insurance at 26%. Generally, private insurance funds provide access to hospitalization services from private providers.[61]

Health insurance schemes are likely to be merely a further means of allowing the private sector to 'facilitate further consolidation of capital at the expense of people's money'. The Government of India policy documents, particularly the Tenth and Eleventh Plans, also recognized the growing inequalities in access to healthcare and the rising out-of-pocket expenditure as a serious concern. The National Health Policy Draft (2015) indicates that inequalities in access need to be addressed through policies that would ensure inclusion of the poor and other vulnerable sections of the population. This in fact pushed the government to develop a stronger contractual arrangement with private sector providers in both the non-profit and for-profit sectors.[62] It also reflected a prevailing ideological view of the potentially greater quality and efficiency of the private sector and the virtues of using competitive contracting as a way of sharing public sector resources. The vision of the neoliberal state proposes that gains from improved management could be obtained within a contracting framework. Hence, the Indian state adopted contract-based models within a publicly set framework and expanded contractual relationships between public and private health sectors. In pursuit of this model, public health budgets have been redirected to subsidize social insurance for those sections of the population (BPL) that have been judged to be unable to pay. Health insurance became one of the viable strategies of the state, which skilfully tried to address both the growing cost of medical care and accessibility concerns.[63]

The High-Level Expert Group (HLEG) report made a departure from the global discourse in suggesting that enhanced public spending on health to 2.5 per cent of GDP should be largely devoted towards strengthening public systems. It also recommended against insurance mechanisms and called for bringing different government insurance programmes under the same umbrella. It rejected insurance sighting the evidence that the bulk of out-of-pocket expenditure (OOPE) was in out-patient services and on drugs and diagnostics. Instead, the HLEG suggested that a national health package would be provided as a guarantee to all citizens and services would be jointly provided by the public sector and the private sector. It suggested two models to engage the private sector: one is the 'coordinated care model' based on public provisioning complemented by contracted-in the private sector; the other is more like a 'managed care model' where private and public facilities would be part of a network to provide health services to empanelled citizens. In this model primary, secondary and tertiary care would be managed as a network, with payments made to the network per person registered. Over the years the corporate health sector, though very few in absolute numbers, has really penetrated the big cities. These are large establishments with huge bed strengths. Apart from these, there are small establishments in the form of nursing homes providing a wide range of secondary care services. But the large majority are still individual practitioners. Between 2000–2001 and 2006–2007 more than 40,000 new establishments have come up, largely in the urban areas. At the same time, small enterprises have almost gone down. These clearly point out that a rapid transformation towards organized forms of production is taking place in urban areas of the country. Parallelly there was also the disappearance of general practitioners who are being included in the medico industrial complex. Given the assurance from the government about cashless services, a lot of people would tend to enrol them with the better looking secondary and tertiary care institutions wherever they are available. In order to incentivize the growth process further, the Government of India has included the health sector in the Viability Gap Funding scheme under which 20 per cent of expenses would be borne by the government if hospitals and medical colleges are set up in non-metros. This, coupled with the market guarantee mechanisms provided under the 'managed care' model, can create conditions for further expansion of the private sector.[64]

Another major development towards the growth of the corporate health sector was the introduction of a new Drug Price Control Order (DPCO) in 1994. Initially, 166 bulk drugs and their formulations were under price control, and the DPCO1995 brought down the number of essential bulk drugs too. The pharmaceutical sector was further liberalized in 2002. The impact of these drug policy changes could be seen in the spiralling increase in drug prices during the period 1994–2004. The overall reforms in the health sector during this period were piecemeal but incremental, which led to extensive changes in the organizational structure, financing and delivery of healthcare services.[65]

Role of Indian Entrepreneurs

In India the growth of the middle classes is not restricted to urban areas; in several states, there has been a rise in the middle and upper middle classes in rural areas as well. This process began with the growth of capitalism in agriculture, surpluses from which were invested in a number of commercial activities including health services. This was seen in Andhra Pradesh, Maharashtra and Gujarat, where families belonging to the rich and middle peasantry made use of public investment in education as a vehicle for social mobility and invested it in educating their children to become professionals. From these prosperous areas, some emigrated to the UK and the US as qualified professionals during the late 1960s and 1970s. A few of them returned to India during the 1980s and set up corporate hospitals in Andhra Pradesh, Tamil Nadu and Gujarat. This in a sense represented the rise of the globalized middle class that put pressure on the government to provide concessions and subsidies to set up corporate hospitals. Anji Reddy (1941–2013) is the founder of Dr Reddy's Laboratories, and Prathap Chandra Reddy (b.1933) is the founder of the Apollo Hospital Chain. Apollo Hospital was the first corporate hospital in India, established in 1984, which was greeted with curiosity and measured relief by the rising middle classes since it brought in a new definition of quality with its corporate management and modern diagnostics. From then on, the growth of private healthcare has been unstoppable: starting with tertiary hospitals, it seamlessly expanded to secondary care, medical and nursing education and diagnostic centres and laboratories. Yusuf Hamied (b.1936) the son of the founder of Cipla, established one of the top five generic drug producers. These individuals are closely connected with two related spheres of action: private hospitals and generic pharmaceutical production.[66]

Notes

1 See Purendra Prasad, "Health Care Reforms: Do They Ensure Social Protection for the Labouring Poor?" And Rama V. Baru, "Medical Industrial Complex: Trends in Corporatization of Health Services", in *Equity and Access: Health Care Studies in India*, ed. Purendra Prasad and Amar Jessani (New Delhi: OUP, 2018).
2 Duggal, *Private Health Care Sector.*
3 Baru, *Private Health Care in India*, 51.
4 Ibid.
5 Sunil Nandaraj, "Beyond the Law and the Lord, Quality of Private Health Care", *Economic and Political Weekly* XXIX, no. 27 (1994): 1680.
6 Ibid.
7 Government of India, Central Bureau of Health Intelligence, *Health Information of India* (New Delhi: Ministry of Health and Family Welfare, various years).
8 Central Bureau of Health Intelligence, *Directory of Hospitals in India, 1985 and 1988* (New Delhi: Ministry of Health and Family Welfare, Government of India).
9 Rama Devi, *Practices of Doctors in Some Government Hospitals in Hyderabad*, Unpublished MPhil Dissertation, University of Hyderabad, 1985, in Baru, *Private Health Care in India*, 51.
10 Ibid.
11 Rama V. Baru, "Privatisation of Health Services, South Asian Perspectives", *Economic and Political Weekly* 38, no. 42 (2003): 4433–37 (Hereafter cited as Baru, "Privatisation of Health Services").
12 Debabar Bannerji, "Landmarks in the Development of Health Services in India", in *Public Health and Poverty of Reforms*, ed. Imrana Qadeer, Kasturi Sen, and K.R. Nayar (New Delhi: Sage Publications, 2001), 44.
13 Ibid., 45.
14 Ibid.
15 Baru, "Privatisation of Health Services", 4434.
16 Rao, *Do We Care?*, 17.
17 Paul Gertler and Van der Jacques Gaag, *Willingness to Pay: Evidence from Two Developing Countries* (Washington, DC: World Bank Publication, 1990), 1.
18 A. Twaddle, "Health Systems Reforms – Toward a Framework for International Comparisons", *Social Science and Medicine* 43, no. 5 (1996): 637–54.

19 I. Gough, *The Political Economy of the Welfare State* (London: Macmillan, 1996) and A. Twaddle, "Health Systems Reforms – Toward a Framework for International Comparisons", *Social Science and Medicine* 43, no. 5 (1996): 637–54.
20 Rao, *Do We Care?*, 53.
21 Rural Health Statistics Bulletin, (2017–2018), Government of India, Ministry of Health and Family Welfare Statistics Division.
22 Rama V. Baru, *Private Health Care in India: Social Characteristics and Trends* (New Delhi: Sage Publications, 1998) and M. Price, "Explaining Trends in the Privatisation of Health Services in South Africa", *Health Policy and Planning* 4, no. 2 (1989): 50–62. See also Gertler and Jacques, *Willingness to Pay*, 2.
23 Government of India, Ministry of Health and Family Welfare, Health Information of India, Central Bureau of Health Intelligence (New Delhi: Govt of India, various years).
24 Shailender Kumar Hooda, "Private Sector in Healthcare Delivery Market in India: Structure, Growth and Implications", *Working Paper 185* (New Delhi: Institute for Studies in Industrial Development, 2015), 7 (Hereafter cited as Hooda, "Private Sector in Healthcare Delivery").
25 S. Sehgal and S. Hooda, "Emerging Role of Private Sector in Indian Health Care Delivery Market: Trends, Pattern and Implications", *Intern Report* (New Delhi: Institute for Studies in Industrial Development (ISID), 2015).
26 Government of India, "Report of Sixth Economic Census", *Ministry of Statistics and Programme Implementation* (Central Statistical Office, 2016).
27 *Health on the March* (2005–2006).
28 *Health on the March* (2018).
29 *Health on the March* (several years).
30 *Health on the March* (2005–2006).
31 *Health on the March* (2018).
32 P.K. Rana and B.P. Mishra, "Ailing Health Status in West Bengal Critical Analysis", *Journal of Law, Policy and Globalization* 2 (2012): 1–7.
33 Ibid.
34 Ibid.
35 Koushik Kumar Hati and Rajarshi Majumdar, "Health for Development: A District Level Study in West Bengal". *MPRA Paper No. 45849* (September 2011).
36 Ibid.
37 West Bengal Development Report, Planning Commission, Government of India (New Delhi: Academic Foundation, 2010). Also see Sandip Kumar Ray, Subhra S. Basu, and Amal Kumar Basu, "An Assessment of Rural Health Care Delivery System in Some Areas of West Bengal — An Overview", *Indian Journal of Public Health* 55, no. 2 (2011); Arijita Dutta, Arpita Ghose, Satarupa Bandyopadhyay, Aniruddha Mukherjee, and B.R. Satpathi, "Hospital Efficiency in West Bengal: A Study on Secondary level Hospital", Funded by Department of Health and Family Welfare Government of West Bengal (2011).
38 Zakir Husain, Saswata Ghosh, and Bijoya Roy, "Socio Economic Profile of Patients in Kolkata: A Case Study of RG Kar and AMRI", *Occasional Paper,* Institute of Development Studies (July 2008), 25.
39 Ibid.
40 Ibid.
41 For details of the rural healthcare conditions in Birbhum, see *The Pratichi Health Report*, Number 1, Pratichi India Trust, 2005.
42 *Seventeenth Report of the Standing Committee on Health and Family Welfare, 1999–2000*; Twelfth Legislative Assembly, Report on Pre-Voting Budget Scrutiny (2000–2001), West Bengal Legislative Assembly Secretariat.
43 Ibid.
44 *West Bengal Human Development Report 2004* (Development and Planning Department, Government of West Bengal, 2004), 136.

45 https://ccs.in › internship_papers › Waiting-for-H … Accessed on 28.05.2010.
46 Ibid. Also see Anirban Ray, "Baro Rajyer Madhye Daktarer sanhkya talanite pashchim-bange", (Number of doctors are miserably poor in this state, compared to other large states) *Ei Samay*, 7 August 2018.
47 G.P. Sandilya, *Medicare: Problems and Remedies* (Kolkata: Basanti Das, 1995), 1.
48 www.financialexpress.com/healthcarebengals/48999/ Accessed on 12.3.2010.
49 Ibid., 2–3.
50 Ibid.
51 Ibid.
52 Tim Lang, "The New Globalisation, Food and Health", in *Health and Disease: A Reader*, ed. Basiro Davey, Alastair Gray, and Clive Seale (Buckingham and Philadelphia: Open University Press, 2002) cited in Imrana Qadeer, "Universal Health Care: The Trojan Horse of Neoliberal Policies", *Social Change* 43 (June 2013): 149–64 (Hereafter cited as Qadeer, "Universal Health Care: The Trojan Horse of Neoliberal Policies").
53 Prabhat Patnaik, A note on the political economy of the 'retreat of the state' in *Whatever Happened to Imperialism and Other Essays* (New Delhi: Tulika, 1995), 195–219 cited in Qadeer, "Universal Health Care: The Trojan Horse of Neoliberal Policies".
54 Roger Jeffery, "Commercialisation in Health Service", in *Global Health Governance and Commercialisation of Public Health in India: Actors, Institutions and Dialectics of Global and Local,* ed. Anuj Kapilashrami and Rama V. Baru (UK: Routledge, 2019), 80–81 (Hereafter cited as Jeffery, "Commercialisation in Health Service"). Also see Indranil Mukhopadhyay, "Universal Health Coverage: The New Face of Neoliberalism", *Social Change* 43 (2013): 177.
55 Baru, "Medical-Industrial Complex", cited in *Equity and Access: Health Care Studies in India*, ed. Purendra Prasad and Amar Jessani (New Delhi: OUP, 2018), 81.
56 Qadeer, "Universal Health Care: The Trojan Horse of Neoliberal Policies", 149–64.
57 Ibid.
58 Carlota Perez, *Technological Revolution and Financial Capital: The Dynamics of Bubbles and Golden Ages* (Cheltenham, UK: Edward Elgar, 2002), cited in Qadeer, "Universal Health Care: The Trojan Horse of Neoliberal Policies", 149–64.
59 Qadeer, "Universal Health Care: The Trojan Horse of Neoliberal Policies", 149–64.
60 Ibid.
61 Sathia Suthanthiraveeran, "The Five Year Plans in India: Overview of Public Health Policies" (researchgate.net). Accessed on 19.10.2021.
62 Sarah Hodges and Mohan Rao, eds., *Public Health and Private Wealth: Stem Cells, Surrogates and Other Strategic Bodies* (New Delhi: Oxford University Press, 2016) cited in Purendra Prasad, "Health Care Reforms: Do They Ensure Social Protection for the Labouring Poor"?
63 Purendra Prasad, "Health Care Reforms: Do They Ensure Social Protection for the Labouring Poor?" And Rama V. Baru, "Medical Industrial Complex: Trends in Corporatization of Health Services", in *Equity and Access: Health Care Studies in India*, ed. Purendra Prasad and Amar Jessani (New Delhi: OUP, 2018), 34. Also see Jeffery, "Commercialisation in Health Service"; Indranil Mukhopadhyay, "Universal Health Coverage: The New Face of Neoliberalism", *Social Change* 43 (2013): 177.
64 Indranil Mukhopadhyay, "Universal Health Coverage: The New Face of Neoliberalism", *Social Change* 43 (2013): 177–90. Also see Hooda, "Health System in Transition in India", 509–10.
65 Baru, "Privatisation of Health Services", 4433. Also see Hooda, "Health System in Transition in India".
66 Baru, "Privatisation of Health Services", 4437; Rao, *Do We Care?*. For details of the life and work of three pharmaceutical entrepreneurs see Jeffery, "Commercialisation in Health Service", in *Global Health Governance and Commercialisation of Public Health in India: Actors, Institutions and Dialectics of Global and Local*, ed. Kapilashrami Anuj and Rama V. Baru (UK: Routledge, 2019).

References

Anirban Ray. "Baro Rajyer Madhye Daktarer sanhkya talanite pashchimbange" (Number of doctors are miserably poor in this state, compared to other large states). Ei Samay, 7 August 2018.

Baru, Rama V. *Private Health Care in India: Social Characteristics and Trends*. New Delhi: Sage Publications, 1998.

Baru, Rama V. "Privatisation of Health Services, South Asian Perspectives". *Economic and Political Weekly* 38, no. 42 (2003): 4433–4437.

Dutta, Arijita, Arpita Ghose, Satarupa Bandyopadhyay, Aniruddha Mukherjee, and B.R. Satpathi. "Hospital Efficiency in West Bengal: A Study on Secondary Level Hospital". Funded by Department of Health and Family Welfare Government of West Bengal, 2011.

Gertler, Paul, and Van der Jacques Gaag. *Willingness to Pay: Evidence from Two Developing Countries*. Washington, DC: World Bank Publication, 1990.

Gough, I. *The Political Economy of the Welfare State*. London: Macmillan, 1996.

Government of India, Central Bureau of Health Intelligence. *Directory of Hospitals in India, 1985 and 1988*. New Delhi: Ministry of Health and Family Welfare, 1988.

Government of India, Central Bureau of Health Intelligence. *Health Information of India*. New Delhi: Ministry of Health and Family Welfare (2005–2010)

Government of India. *Report of Sixth Economic Census. Ministry of Statistics and Programme Implementation*. New Delhi: Central Statistical Office, 2016.

Government of India. *Rural Health Statistics Bulletin (2017–2018)*. New Delhi: Ministry of Health and Family Welfare Statistics Division, 2018.

Government of India. *West Bengal Development Report*. New Delhi: Planning Commission, Academic Foundation, 2010.

Government of West Bengal. *Directorate of Health Services, State Bureau of Health Intelligence, Health on the March*. Calcutta, (1967–1972).

Government of West Bengal. *West Bengal Human Development Report, 2004*. Kolkata: Development and Planning Department, 2004.

Hooda, Shailender Kumar. "Private Sector in Healthcare Delivery Market in India: Structure, Growth and Implications". *Working Paper* 185. New Delhi: Institute for Studies in Industrial Development, 2015.

Hooda, Shailendra. "Health System in Transition in India: Journey from State Provisioning to Privatization". *World Review of Political Economy* 11, no. 4 (Winter 2020): 63–84.

https://www.ccs.in/internship_papers/2008/Waiting-for-Healthcare-A-survey-of-a-public-hospital-in-Kolkata-Mansi.pdf

Hussain, Zakir, Saswata Ghosh, and Bijoya Roy. "Socio Economic Profile of Patients in Kolkata: A Case Study of RG Kar and AMRI". *Occasional Paper*. Institute of Development Studies, Kolkata, July 2008.

Kapilashrami, Anuj, and Rama V. Baru, eds. *Global Health Governance and Commercialisation of Public Health in India: Actors, Institutions and Dialectics of Global and Local*. London and New York: Routledge, 2019.

Kumar Rana. *The Pratichi Health Report*, Number 1, Kolkata: Pratichi India Trust, 2005.

Mukhopadhyay, Indranil. "Universal Health Coverage: The New Face of Neoliberalism". *Social Change* 43 (2013): 177–190.

Nandaraj, Sunil. "Beyond the Law and the Lord, Quality of Private Health Care". *Economic and Political Weekly* XXIX, no. 27 (1994): 1680–1685.

Prasad, Purendra, and Amar Jessani, eds. *Equity and Access: Health Care Studies in India.* New Delhi: OUP, 2018.

Price, M. "Explaining Trends in the Privatisation of Health Services in South Africa". *Health Policy and Planning* 4, no. 2 (1989): 121–130.

Qadeer, Imrana. "Universal Health Care: The Trojan Horse of Neoliberal Policies". *Social Change* 43 (June 2013): 149–164.

Qadeer, Imrana, Kasturi Sen, and K.R. Nayar, eds. *Public Health and Poverty of Reforms.* New Delhi: Sage Publications, 2001.

Rana, Koushik Kumar, and Rajarshi Majumdar. "Health for Development: A District Level Study in West Bengal". *MPRA Paper Number* 45849 (September 2011).

Rao, K. Sujatha. *Do We Care? India's Health System.* New Delhi: OUP, 2020.

Ray, Sandip Kumar, Subhra S. Basu, and Amal Kumar Basu. "An Assessment of Rural Health Care Delivery System in Some Areas of West Bengal — An Overview". *Indian Journal of Public Health* 55, no. 2 (2011): 70–80.

Sandilya, G.P. *Medicare: Problems and Remedies.* Kolkata: Basanti Das, 1995.

Sehgal, S., and S. Hooda. "Emerging Role of Private Sector in Indian Health Care Delivery Market: Trends, Pattern and Implications". *Intern Report*, New Delhi: Institute for Studies in Industrial Development (ISID), 2015.

Suthanthiraveeran, Sathia. "The Five Year Plans in India: Overview of Public Health Policies". researchgate.net, 2011.

Twaddle, A. "Health Systems Reforms – Toward a Framework for International Comparisons". *Social Science and Medicine* 43, no. 5 (1996): 637–654.

West Bengal Legislative Assembly Secretariat. *Seventeenth Report of the Standing Committee on Health and Family Welfare, 1999–2000.* Twelfth Legislative Assembly, Report on Pre-Voting Budget Scrutiny (2000–2001).

www.financialexpress.com/healthcarebengals/48999/.

5 The Metamorphosis of Private Healthcare

Introduction

The discussion so far has focused on the drive towards developing a vibrant private healthcare sector in India and West Bengal (Kolkata) under local as well as global compulsions. It is obvious that neither the decline of the public healthcare sector nor the development of the private healthcare sector should be studied in a simple cause and effect relation structure. Several other factors have contributed to the growth of the latter, but these two phenomena are closely interlinked with each other. The global pressure of investing more in private healthcare and reforming the degenerating public healthcare services brought about far-reaching consequences in the entire healthcare culture of the metropolis. The dependence upon the market forces and the techno-centric approach to health strengthened the significance and the expansion of private healthcare. Actually, the allocation on healthcare had always been meagre compared to the demand of the vast population in India. Since this inadequate infrastructure failed to come up with positive outcomes, it collapsed after three decades of Independence, providing the space for the private health sector to flourish as the alternative for healthcare delivery services. Further decay was brought about by the shrinking of the welfare state towards the provisioning of funds for the healthcare sector. This aggravated the failure of the public healthcare services and cleared the subsequent rise of the private health sector. This process received a boom in the post-liberalization era with the coming of the international donor agencies with a new package of reforms for public healthcare and the thrust towards developing the private healthcare sector.

The aim of this chapter is to focus on the impact of the growth of the private healthcare sector. Along with this, the changing nature, characteristics, size and utilization pattern of this sector in the post-liberalization era with special reference to Kolkata will be discussed. It will also discuss the reforms that were undertaken in the public hospitals and their subsequent impact on the health services. Attempts will be made to unravel the effects of the growing dominance of the private healthcare sector which converted healthcare into a commodity and increased the cases of medical negligence and malpractice. The changes in the entire healthcare culture have indeed 'medicalized' life to its fullest and created an atmosphere of sickness where the normal human beings are always under the

DOI: 10.4324/9781003169475-6

threat of being ill. These changes not only intensified the crisis of the delivery of healthcare services but also challenged the accessibility of nominal healthcare for the population at large.

Neoliberal Phase in Health Sector: From Private to Corporate

The corporatization of health services and the consolidation of markets within it is an important feature of the Indian healthcare economy from the 1990s onwards. The concept of commercialization acknowledges the role of markets within and outside the public sector. It emphasizes

> the provision of health care services through market relationships to those able to pay; investment in, and production of those services, and of inputs to them, for cash income or profit, including private contracting and supply to publicly financed health care; and health care finance from individual payments and private insurance.[1]

On the other hand, White[2] has defined 'Corporatization' of healthcare to describe the penetration of large for-profit companies into an area previously dominated by non-profit institutions and individual practitioners. It also refers to certain organizational-managerial reforms of public services adopted under the aegis of the World Bank, such as application of management practices of the corporate sector to public hospitals with the understanding that this will improve their efficiency and hence the effectiveness of public expenditures.

The consolidation and transformation of markets in the Indian health service system present the features of medical industrial complex. Drawing on the analogy of the military-industrial complex, Arnold Relman, the former editor of *The New England Journal of Medicine*, characterized the rise of diverse business interests in medicine as a medical industrial complex in the USA during the 1980s. He along with several others who were critical of private interests in medical care wrote extensively on the entrenched network of power relations, the rise of business lobbies and their influence on policy. Capital consolidated itself in medical services through pharmaceutical, medical devices, insurance and provisioning corporations in the USA. Public health reforms were diluted during the Clinton and Obama regimes and the interests of corporate American medical care remained largely protected.[3] This similar pattern is also reflected in the development of healthcare service in the post-reform phase.

President and CEO of GE Healthcare India has observed that India is the first country to have a large number of multinational healthcare providers. There are seven to eight very active MNCs. It opens a whole host of opportunities.[4] Increasingly over the past decade, there is strong advocacy and promotion by the industry of the idea that 'Health care infrastructure should not just be viewed as a social good but also as a viable economic venture with productivity'.[5] The Confederation of Indian Industry (CII) projects healthcare sector as one with immense importance for the national economy, due to its rising contribution to

GDP and the potential to be an engine of growth for the nation as it can create '70 to 80 million jobs in the next 10 year.' The CII National Healthcare Division, comprising hospitals, diagnostic centres, and medical equipment companies, regularly organizes the India Health Summit since 2002 to promote private investment in the healthcare sector and lobby for concessions and favourable policies.[6] One of the demands of the Federation of Indian Chambers of Commerce and Industry (FICCI) Health Services Division is that the government should attract private healthcare investment to supplement the public funding deficit in healthcare allocations, by giving various fiscal and non-fiscal incentives.

'Corporatization of healthcare in India: The liberalization effect'[7] gave an excellent overview of the healthcare situation in the post-liberalization era. One of the most significant trends emerging in the wake of liberalization is the new vigour of the entry of corporate hospitals and multinationals in the healthcare scenario. The reason for this new tempo is the potential that India offers to NRIs and multinationals. Since the early 1990s, when healthcare was seen as a 'sunrise industry,' several big corporate houses, Fortis Healthcare (promoted by Ranbaxy Labs), Wockhardt Hospitals (promoted by the pharma company, Wockhardt) and Max Healthcare announced plans to set up hospital chains across the country. In addition to these big hospital chains, including the oldest one Apollo, other private hospitals and specialized healthcare facilities have been created for specialized services such as cardiac care, renal care, eye care, orthodontics, and laparoscopic surgery.[8]

Mention should be made that the International Finance Corporation (IFC), a private sector lending arm of the World Bank, has granted loans to several hospital projects that include Max Healthcare, Rockland, Artemis, Apollo and Duncan Gleneagles. Since 2002, IFC has extended loans to Apollo twice. In June 2009, IFC provided loans amounting to $50 million to Apollo Hospitals Enterprises Limited (AHEL) to expand its Apollo Reach network, specifically to set up smaller hospitals in the next three years in semi-urban and rural areas, in Tier-II cities, to provide 'affordable health care' to low-income populations in these areas, using cross-subsidisation between 'high-income and low-income consumers'. IFC is promoting this activity of AHEL as an 'innovative and inclusive business model'. More recently international private equity firms like AIG, J.P. Morgan Stanley, Carlyle, Blackstone Group, Quantum and Blue Ridge have been investing in hospital projects. In a further sign of international involvement in financing commercial healthcare in India, smaller groups such as Portea (Healthvista India) and Regency (based in Kanpur) have also recently accessed loans (see Table 5.1).[9]

Apollo, Max and Fortis were the three active healthcare groups in India. The Apollo group is reported to be the largest healthcare group in Asia followed by the Fortis group (CRISIL Research 2009). Since 2003 Apollo Hospital Enterprises Ltd (AHEL) has consistently held 30 per cent of the market share, while other healthcare companies were way behind, each holding less than 10 per cent. As has been mentioned earlier Apollo hospital in Chennai not only marks the rise of corporatization of healthcare in India but Dr Prathap Reddy, a cardiologist professional long practising in the USA, returned to India in the late1970s and lobbied with the

Table 5.1 Indian Corporate Hospitals Projects Funded by the International Finance Corporation 1997–2017

Corporation	Project Cost (US$ Millions)	IFC Loan / Investment (US$ Millions)	IFC Input as Percentage of Total Project Cost (%)	Year of Signing
Duncan Gleneagles	29	7	24	1997
Max Healthcare	84	18	21	2002
Apollo Hospitals	70	20	29	2005
Artemis	40	10	25	2006
Max Healthcare	90	67	74	2007
Rockland	76	22	29	2008
Max Healthcare	93	30	32	2009
Apollo Hospitals	200	50	25	2009
Apollo Hospitals	n.s.	60	n.a.	2012
Global Hospitals	60	25	42	2013
Fortis	n.s.	100	n.a.	2013
Portea	37	7	19	2015
Eye-Q	10	5.7	57	2015
Regency	25	9	36	2016
Apollo Hospitals	135	68	50	2016
Glenmark	200	75	38	2016
Granules	84	48	57%	2016
Healthcare Global	n.s.	15	n.a.	2016
Max Healthcare	325	75	23	2017
Biological E	n.s	60	n.a.	2017

Source: www.ifc.org and Lefebvre (2010).[10]

Notes n.s=not Stated; n.a.=not available. The loan in Eye-Q was denominated in Indian rupees; the exchange rate applied was Rs.60=US$1

Indian political class and bureaucracy to create conducive business conditions for corporate hospitals. It is interesting to point out that the real push for liberalizing import duties came from Reddy when he set up the first corporate hospital in India. He modelled the Apollo hospital in the image of an American multispecialty hospital that required high-end equipment like CT scanners which had to be imported. For this Reddy had to get necessary permissions from the central governments. He used social, political and bureaucratic networks to bring about the changes in the import policy for medical equipment. Hodges[11] argued that the climate for liberalization already existed and the political class was ideologically in sync with Reddy's project. Reddy's considerable lobbying with Indira Gandhi and Rajiv Gandhi brought about changes in rules relating to finance and imports. Reddy also lobbied with several ministers and specially acknowledges the role played by Pranab Mukherjee and R. Venkataraman who supported the Apollo project.[12]

AHEL is also into a range of other medical care related services: nursing and hospital management colleges, pharmacies, diagnostic clinics, medical transcription services, telemedicine, clinical trials, and consulting. The Group comprise Apollo Hospitals, Apollo Health and Lifestyle Ltd, Apollo Pharmacy, Apollo

Reach Hospitals, Apollo Hospitals Education and Research Foundation, Apollo Telemedicine Networking Foundation, Apollo Insurance Company Ltd, Apollo DKV a joint venture of Apollo with two of Europe's big insurance groups – DKV AG and a Munich Re Group Company and Apollo Global Projects Consultancy. The Apollo Health care Consulting Services manages more than 30 hospitals in India, Dhaka, Colombo, Kuwait, Nigeria, and Yemen. All such managed hospitals become part of the network for central marketing and purchasing programs. In addition, Apollo also has an Online Hospital Equipment Services Private Ltd (Equipment World), an electronic equipment exchange for medical equipment and high-end medical technology. Apollo Gleneagles is a joint venture between Apollo and Parkway Group of Singapore[13] to cater to eastern and north-eastern India, Bangladesh, Bhutan, Myanmar and Nepal. AHEL has a 45.5 per cent stake in Apollo Health Street, an associated company that provides IT services to US healthcare companies. AHEL through Stem Cell Therapeutics India, in association with Cadila Pharma and Stem Cyte, USA, has set up an umbilical cord blood stem cell banking facility at Ahmedabad, at a total investment of Rs 60 crore.

The Fortis Group, incorporated in 1996, is the healthcare division of Religare Technova, a holding company for the IT business of the diversified transnational Indian business group Ranbaxy. The other divisions include diagnostics (Super Religare Laboratories SRL, formerly SRL Ranbaxy), financial services (Religare Enterprises), wellness, and aviation and travel. In early 2008 Fortis had a network of 13 hospitals primarily in north Indian cities and 16 satellite and heart centres, including one in Afghanistan. By late 2008 it was reported to own 22 hospitals and 2,500 beds of which 1,600 beds were operational. Fortis Healthcare care planned to set up ten 'medicities' and was engaged in talks with the Gujarat government on establishing one such project in that state. In January 2009 Fortis, through its wholly owned subsidiary Novelife Limited, along with a Mauritian Industrial Group CIEL, jointly acquired a controlling stake in Mauritius's largest private hospital. Fortis took over the operations and management of the hospital. As of March 2010, Fortis Healthcare Network comprised 46 hospitals (including 13 satellite/heart centres).[14]

Presently, Fortis Healthcare Limited – an IHH Healthcare Berhad Company – is a leading integrated healthcare services provider in India. It is one of the largest healthcare organizations in the country with 36 healthcare facilities (including projects under development), 4,000 operational beds and over 400 diagnostics centres. Fortis is present in India, United Arab Emirates (UAE) and Sri Lanka. The company is listed on the BSE Ltd and National Stock Exchange (NSE) of India. It draws strength from its partnership with global major and parent company, IHH, to build upon its culture of world-class patient care and superlative clinical excellence. Fortis employs 23,000 people (including SRL) who share its vision of becoming the world's most trusted healthcare network. Fortis offers a full spectrum of integrated healthcare services ranging from clinics to quaternary care facilities and a wide range of ancillary services.[15]

Max India Limited is a multi-business corporate company (part of the Mohan Singh Group). Prior to 2000, Max was in the telecommunications and the traditional manufacturing sector. Seeing an opportunity it shifted to healthcare services. Max Healthcare is owned by its founders and other promoters, Warburg Pincus (reportedly the largest international private equity investor in India), and other foreign institutional investors and individuals. It claims to 'protect life' through its life insurance subsidiary Max New York Life, a joint venture between Max India and New York Life, a Fortune 100 company. It promotes 'care for life' through its healthcare company, Max Healthcare, a subsidiary of Max India Limited. Max Healthcare has a technical collaboration with Partners Harvard Medical International; Max claims to 'enhance life' through its health insurance company, Max Bupa Health Insurance, a joint venture between Max India and Bupa Finance Plc., UK; and finally, it will 'improve life' through its clinical research business, Max Neeman, a fully owned subsidiary of Max India. Max India continues the manufacture of speciality products for the packaging industry. Max Healthcare claims to have over 800 Beds and eight hospitals in Delhi with over 1,500 physicians and 3,000 support staff. Max has received IFC assistance in three phases – in 2003, 2007 and in 2009. In 2007 it received a loan to expand its network of secondary and tertiary facilities by 2010, as well as construct new hospitals in the National Capital Region (comprising Delhi and neighbouring townships) and Dehradun. Max planned to set up 16 primary care centres, five nursing homes (each with 30–40 beds), and two tertiary level hospitals, at a total budget of around Rs 3 billion.[16]

The Wockhardt Hospitals established a chain of so-called 'state-of-the-art super speciality' hospitals located at Nagpur, Nashik, Surat, Rajkot, Bhavnagar, Vashi (Mumbai), Bangalore, Hyderabad and Kolkata.[17]

However, Fortis took over the greenfield hospitals division of Wockhardt Hospitals comprising ten hospitals in metro cities of Mumbai, Bangalore and Kolkata (including two under construction) for Rs 909 crore, on a going-concern basis. The acquisition was made under a wholly-owned subsidiary, Fortis Hospitals and was funded partly by the recently concluded rights issue, internal accruals and debt. The acquisition expanded Fortis' bed capacity by 1,902 (including 534 beds in two under-construction projects) and provided a significant presence in south, west and east India. The aggregate bed capacity of Fortis Network now stands at 5,180. With the addition of the ten Wockhardt Hospitals, Fortis would now have six hospitals in Bangalore, four in Mumbai and three in Kolkata apart from a vast presence in the national capital region and a major facility in Chennai.[18]

Along with these giants investing in healthcare there are also other companies which were pouring their capital into healthcare investments. The table below lists the private hospital chains in India in 2017 (see Table 5.2).

As a result of corporatization, the healthcare industry is reported to be 'flush with private equity (PE) funds'. According to business reports, there has been an increase in PE funding in healthcare. Healthcare companies are reported to prefer PE fund over raising capital through public offers or debt. The investment of PE funds was reported to be taking place not just for established hospital chains in urban areas but also for hospitals in Tier-II and Tier-III cities, rural

Table 5.2 Private Hospital Chains in India in 2017[19]

Hospital Chain	Year of Creation	Base	Number of Hospitals	Number of Beds
Manipal	1953	Bangalore (Kar)	11	2333
Apollo	1983	Chennai (TN)	36	7778
RG stone	1987	Delhi	14	349
Kuval	1987	Coimbatore (TN)	3	857
Wockhardt	1989	Mumbai (Mah)	9	1330
Seven Hills	1992	Visakhapatnam (AP)	2	556
Sahyadri	1993	Pune (Mah)	10	900
VrundavanShalby	1994	Ahmedabad (Guj)	7	640
CARE	1997	Hyderabad (AP)	17	2400
Metro Heart	1997	Delhi	12	1814
Global	1998	Hyderabad (AP)	5	1950
Vikram	2000	Mysore (Kar)	7	329
Sterling	2001	Ahmedabad (Guj)	7	1006
Fortis	2001	Delhi	27	4564
HeallhCare Global	2001	Bangalore (Kar)	13	550
Narayana Hrudayalaya	2001	Bangalore (Kar)	13	6650
Max	2002	Delhi	9	1840
Rockland	2004	Delhi	5	1315
Vaatsalya	2005	Bangalore (Kar)	17	1143
Columbia	2005	Bangalore (Kar)	11	1181
All			230	38909

and semi-urban areas, diagnostic centres and medical equipment. For instance, New York-based Acumen Fund and Hindustan Latex Ltd (HLL, a government enterprise) had formed a joint venture (JV) called Life Spring Hospitals, which was creating a chain of small hospitals (20–25 beds), in UP to provide maternal and child healthcare services for the lower middle-income group in semi-urban areas. ICICI Venture, which floated I-Ven Medicare in mid-2007, had invested in not-so-renowned names in health care. It invested US$36 million in Sahyadri Hospital, Pune; US$24 million in Vikram Hospital, Mysore; US$16.25 million in Medica Synergy, Kolkata; and US$10.25 million in RG Stone, New Delhi. PE firms were also reported to be investing in independent diagnostic centres. For example, ICICI Venture had invested '35 crore in Metropolis Health Services in 2006'. Venture Capital firm Sequoia Capital India had invested $10 million in Dr Lal PathLabs.[20]

Rapid growth of private diagnostic centres is another major development in the field of corporate health sector. Chakravarthy[21] has pointed out several factors which are responsible for the emergence of the number of private diagnostic facilities. The growth of such independent diagnostic facilities is perceived as taking a load off of conventional hospitals. Specialized diagnostic labs are looking at Hospital Lab Management (HLM) — ways by which they could take over the maintenance and operation of lab facilities at big hospitals. This is seen as an avenue for those who do not want to open a new lab or buy one outright. Another development is the government's policy of encouraging/promoting public–private partnerships (PPP) in healthcare. In the context of PPP, laboratory services are being outsourced by government and other public sector hospitals as well as institutions, such as the Railways, Defense, and Employees' State Insurance Corporation. The outsourcing of laboratory testing and diagnostic services by non-Indian hospitals is expected to become a big business in India.

Corporate presence is also seen in the diagnostic facilities. Some of the major companies investing in the diagnostic facilities are SRL, the Mumbai-based Metropolis, the Delhi-based Dr Lal's Pathlabs and the Agarwal Imaging Centre. Pharma companies, including Dr Reddy's Laboratories (DRL) and Nicholas Piramal, entered this field. Metropolis Health Services (India) Private Limited is a Mumbai-based company which runs a chain of clinical diagnostic centres across the country in Mumbai, Chennai, Bangalore, Jaipur, Thrissur, Kochi, Delhi, Ahmedabad and a contact centre at Dubai.[22]

So we can say that there is a huge dominance of the private healthcare sector in its heterogeneous form giving shape to the Indian healthcare industry. In the previous chapter, we have seen that during 2010–2011 the number of private healthcare institutions was approximately 10.4 lakh. With the corporatization of healthcare, the number has multiplied. According to NSSO 2013, 67th round NSS, India had more than 743,000 hospitals, 1,654,000 hospital beds; 72 per cent of hospitals and 60 per cent of beds were in the private sector. Of a total of one million private healthcare enterprises, about 25 per cent were medium to large medical establishments. The rest were microenterprises. However, the share of informal medical practitioners decreased with the rapid rise of the bigger and formal sector practitioners/enterprises. Estimates from Economic Survey 2016 reveal that around four-fifths of the total number (983,018) of health enterprises were private. Private partnerships and private companies, as well as cooperative enterprises, are large relative to others in terms of the number of health workers they employ. This indicates that the majority of large hospitals are of a private corporate/company nature. According to a Services Sector Enterprises Survey by the NSS (National Sample Survey), the private sector consisted of 10.67 lakh private providers, ranging from informal to large formal and corporate entities, as opposed to a low 1.96 lakh public hospitals/centres. The growth pattern of the private sector reveals that the private sector grew at a much faster rate during the liberalization and privatization policy reforms, a period that saw a number of tax benefits and other incentives provided for setting up private hospitals/clinics. Estimates from a different round of NSS research reveal that large/corporate hospitals are growing/emerging rapidly, while small providers are vanishing over time – a phenomenon of big fish eating smaller fish. That is, large healthcare providers are growing at a faster rate, indicating a rapid shift towards an organized form of healthcare delivery, particularly in urban areas. The present growth pattern seems to favour a kind of private healthcare market that is concentrated in fewer hands. Smaller providers and individual practitioners in these areas are getting sucked into large and corporate-run hospital networks that create further induced demand. This means that the increasing corporatization of the healthcare market in the country is proving beneficial for healthcare providers.[23]

In a recent study by the Centre for Disease Economics and Policies (India) and Princeton University,[24] it has been shown that India has approximately 1.9 million hospital beds, 95,000 ICU beds and 48,000 ventilators. Nationally, hospital beds are concentrated in the private sector (hospital beds: 1,185,242 private vs 713,986 public). ICU beds and ventilators follow a similar trend (ICU beds: 59,262 private vs 35,699 public; ventilators: 29,631 private: 17,850 public).

Utilization Pattern

The access to health services appears to be a key mechanism for better health outcomes (see Table 5.3). The central role of high utilization rates has major policy implications. It confirms the need to ensure access to health services and to focus on interventions that will improve utilization of health facilities. It also highlights the need to promote behavioural changes that will motivate people to seek appropriate care when ill. Due to its high dominance in the area of service provision, the private sector also became dominant in-service delivery both for inpatient as well as outpatient care services. In 2014, around two-thirds of inpatient and three-quarters of outpatient care treatments were received from the private sector. The outpatient care treatment received from the private sector, however, has been almost constant since 1986–1987, but in providing inpatient treatments its share increased to 68 per cent in urban and 58 per cent in rural in 2014 from a low share of 40 per cent in 1986–1987 (see Table 5.3).

Foreign Direct Investment (FDI)

This liberalized regulatory framework provides considerable scope for foreign direct investment in India's healthcare sector, i.e., in hospitals and diagnostic centres, through various modes of financing. Specifically, these liberal policies permit international investments in Indian hospitals through FDI, foreign institutional investment (FII), venture capital (VC) funds, private equity (PE) funds, initial placement offers (IPOs) subscribed to by foreign players and non-resident Indians (NRI). It was held that FDI provides the much-needed resources to

Table 5.3 Inpatient and Outpatient Care Treatments by Type of Facilities (in %)[25]

		Inpatient		Outpatient	
		Public	Private	Public	Private
42nd: 1986–1987	Total	60.0	40.0	22.5	77.5
52nd: 1995–1996	Total	43.5	56.6	19.5	80.5
60th: 2005–2005	Total	40.0	60.1	20.5	79.5
71st: 2014	Rural	41.9	58.1	28.9	71.1
	Urban	32.0	68.0	21.2	78.8

accelerate capital formation, facilitates transfer of technology, knowledge skills and organizational and managerial capabilities, provides access to international market networks, and so on. Foreign Direct Investment (FDI) is perceived as a magic wand that will transform India into an advanced nation with modern infrastructure. In the process of liberalization and globalization, the government has introduced various policy changes in order to attract FDI in different sectors. In order to promote foreign players, the Government of India raised the FDI cap in the hospital sector to 100 per cent under automatic route in January 2000. With this liberalized rule, for the last one and a half decade, the government has been actively engaged in building a positive economic climate for the healthcare industry. Measures taken include reduction in direct taxes, permitting higher rate of depreciation of medical equipment, income tax exemptions for five years for rural hospitals, custom duty exemptions for imported lifesaving equipments, income tax exemption for health insurance, and active engagement through publicly financed health insurance, which now covers almost 27 per cent of the population. An analysis of the total FDI equity inflow into the hospital sector (hospitals and diagnostic centres) out of total FDI inflow into the healthcare sector (that comprises three sectors like drugs and pharmaceuticals; hospitals and diagnostic centres; medical and surgical appliances) shows that it constitutes a small share (around 21 per cent) of the total share during the period from January 2000 to December 2013.[26]

Following companies undertook the collaborative ventures:[27]

- Singapore's Pacific Healthcare has made its foray into the Indian market, opening an international medical centre, which is a joint venture with India's Vitae Healthcare, in Hyderabad.
- The Singapore-based Parkway Group Healthcare PTE Ltd penetrated into the Indian health care market in 2003 through a joint venture with the Apollo group to build the Apollo Gleneagles hospital, a 325-bed multi-speciality hospital at a cost of US$ 29 million.
- Columbia Asia Group, a Seattle-based hospital services company, a worldwide developer and operator of community hospitals, has started its first American-style medical centre in Hebbal, Bangalore. Columbia Asia is the first hospital to enter the Indian healthcare market through the Foreign Direct Investment route.
- Wockhardt, the international arm of the Harvard Medical School, which also has a strategic association with Harvard Medical International, has set up a new hospital (a tertiary service provider) in Bangalore at a cost of around Rs 200 crore.
- The Parkway Group has also entered into a joint venture with Mumbai-based Asian Heart Institute and Research Centre to set up specialized centres of medical excellence in Mumbai.
- Max Healthcare and Singapore General Hospital (SGH) have entered into collaboration for medical practice, research, training and education in healthcare services.

- Steris, a US$ 1.1 billion healthcare equipment company, has set up a wholly-owned arm in India to sell its devices and products in the country's booming medical device market.
- Apollo Hospitals Enterprise Ltd has entered into a joint venture with Amcare Labs, an affiliate of Johns Hopkins International of the USA, to set up a diagnostic laboratory in Hyderabad.
- India's first geriatric hospital, the Heritage Hospital of Hyderabad has formed a joint venture with US-based United Church Homes to recruit, train and provide placement to registered Indian nurses in the USA.
- The US-based healthcare products major, Proton Health Care has made an entry into India with its range of digital health monitoring devices and has a strategic tie-up with the Delhi-based S.M. Logistics for distributing its products in the Indian market.
- The American Association of Physicians of Indian Origin (AAPI), a Non-Resident Indian group, has been running rural healthcare projects in various Indian states. It had entered into a memorandum of understanding with the Government of India in this regard.

In order to understand the extent and nature of foreign direct investment in hospitals, we obtained a list of all FDI-approved projects in hospitals and diagnostic centres between January 2000 and July 2006 from the Department for Industrial Policy and Promotion. This list consisted of 90 projects, for a total approved FDI amount of $53 million, and covering a wide range of countries, such as Australia, Canada, UK, US, the UAE, Malaysia and Singapore, among others. However, the majority of these approved projects are diagnostic centres. Only 21 of the approved projects are in the hospitals segment. The following table shows the approved projects for FDI in hospitals as received from the DIPP, along with the source countries, and the Rupee and US dollar values of FDI approved.[28] (see Table 5.4).

However, it is important to note that the share of FDI equity inflow to the hospital sector shows increasing trends over the period. Its share increased from 13 per cent during 2000–2005 to around 25.5 per cent in 2013, though subject to year-to-year fluctuations. This reflects that owing to the liberalized foreign investment framework, a significant number of multinational players have been focusing on the Indian hospital sector and have enlarged their presence through partnerships and investments in joint venture projects.[30]

India improved its Ease of Doing Business ranking from 142 in 2014 to 63 in 2019, a jump of 79 positions. India has also been ranked number 1 in the Central and South Asian region in the Global Innovation Index, an improvement of 33 positions, from number 81 globally in 2015 to number 48 in 2020. India has been one of the fastest-growing emerging economies over the last two decades, receiving large FDI inflows, which have grown from US$2.5 billion in 2000–2001 to US$50 billion in 2019–2020. In health, FDI has been concentrated in pharmaceuticals, constituting approximately two-thirds of the total health-sector-related FDI

Table 5.4 Approved FDI Hospitals by DIPP (January 2000–June 2006)[29]

Sl. No.	Date	Indian Company	Country of Foreign Investor	Foreign Equity (Millions)	
				Rs	**US$**
1	April 2002	Fernandez Maternity Hospital, Hyderabad	Australia	0.42	0.01
2	December 2002	Sir Edward Dunlop Hospitals. New Delhi	Canada	1.282.25	26.71
3	January 2004	Max Healthcare. New Delhi	Mauritius	316.21	6.63
4	January 2000	Dr. Ramayya's Pramila Hospitals Ltd. Hyderabad	UK-NRI	15.00	0.35
5	January 2000	HN Hospital. Mumbai	USA- XR]	0.00	0.00
6	September 2003	KalingaHospital, Bhubaneshwar	NRI	54.09	0.11
7	August 2000	Thaqdees Hospitals Ltd, Thaikkatukkara, Kerala	Saudi Arabia	0.32	0.01
8	1 January 2003	Duncan Gleneagles, Kolkata	Singapore	59.24	1.29
9	July 2004	Pacific Hospitals, Hyderabad	Singapore	5.82	0.13
10	October 2001	Malabar Institute of Medical Sciences Hospital Ltd., Calicut	UAE	133.01	2.97
11	July 2002	Peoples General Hospital Ltd. Bhopal	UAE	73.32	1.53
12	August 2001	Thaqdees Hospitals Ltd, Ernakulam	UK	0.34	0.01
13	July 2001	Trichur Heart Hospital. Thrissur"	UK	49.89	1.11
14	August 2002	Bhimavaram Hospital Ltd., Bhimavaram	USA	0.10	0.00
15	December 2002	S&V Loga Hospital Pvt. Ltd, Peramanur, Salem	USA	3.79	0.08
16	November 2003	Vikram Hospital, Mysore	USA	29.05	0.64
17	February 2004	Basappa Memorial Hospital Pvt .Ltd., Mysore	USA	22.83	0.50
18	April 2004	Parekh Hospital Pvt. Ltd. Mumbai	USA	0.50	0.01
19	July 2004	Columbia Asia Hospital Pvt. Ltd., Bangalore	USA	0.90	0.02
20	August 2004	Add Life Medical Institute Ltd. Sterling Hospital Building, Ahmadabad	USA	326.24	7.07
21	January 2004	RA Multispecialty Hospital Pvt. Ltd, Coimbatore	British Virginia	0.06	0.00

over the last two decades. Thus, there is considerable scope for more FDI in the medical devices manufacturing segment, in particular, for discouraging import dependency. FDI in India's health sector (2000–2020) amounts to US$25,357 million. In drug and pharmaceuticals, it is US$16,501 million, in hospital and diagnostic centres, it amounts to US$6,727 million and in medical and surgical appliances it is US$2,130 million. The healthcare sector has received heightened interest from investors (venture capital and private equity) over the last few years, with the transaction value increasing from US$94 million (2011) to US$1,275 million (2016) – a jump of over 13.5 times. Initial Public Offerings (IPOs) of four major companies, Dr Lal Path Labs, HCG, Narayana Hrudayalaya and Thyrocare were oversubscribed, reinforcing investor confidence in the sector. A slew of investments by global health players, including the Parkway Group and a host of players from the Middle East, have strengthened the perception of India as an attractive healthcare investment destination.[31]

Moreove, mention may be made that Indian medical devices market stood at Rs 77,539 crore (US$ 11 billion) in 2020. The market is expected to increase at a compound annual growth rate (CAGR of 35.4 per cent from 2020 to 2025, reaching Rs 352,450 crore (US$ 50 billion)[32]

Pharmaceutical Industries

Ranbaxy, Cipla, Dr Reddy's and other large Indian pharmaceuticals companies have continued to grow, along with the personal wealth of the founder's families. In September 2015, a large section gained their wealth from the pharmaceutical sector.[33] There are over 10,500 manufacturing units and 3,000 pharma companies in India. Over 60,000 generic brands exist across 60 therapeutic categories. India accounts for 20 per cent of global exports in generics, making it the largest provider of generic medicines globally. Indian vaccines are exported to 150 countries. Drugs worth US$130 billion are expected to go off-patent between FY17 to FY22 (Financial Year), presenting a huge market opportunity for Indian manufacturers. With increasing penetration of chemists, especially in rural India, OTC drugs will be readily available. Pharma companies have increased spending to tap rural markets and develop better infrastructure. The market share of hospitals increased from 13.1 per cent in 2009 to 26 per cent in 2020. Over US$200 billion is to be spent on medical infrastructure in the next decade. Following the introduction of product patents, several multinational companies are expected to launch patented drugs in India. India's cost of production is significantly lower than that of the USA and almost half of that of Europe. India's total exports of pharmaceuticals (APIs, generics and alternative system of medicine) during 2016–2017 was US$16.8 billion. India has a market share of almost 42 per cent of generic drugs produced globally, a market size of Africa and the Middle East put together. North America is India's largest export market, receiving over 34 per cent of India's pharmaceuticals exports.[34] The owners of Ranbaxy, Cipla and Dr Reddy share the common characteristics of having built companies that are now able to produce medicines in very large quantities and at considerable profit, and with an international reach, owning companies in Europe and America.[35] Table 5.5 will show how the Indian pharmaceutical companies incurred wealth from the health sector.

Thus, it can be inferred that the intrusion of global capital in the form of FDI in the hospitals of India not only strengthened the market for the private healthcare sector, it has also played a pivotal role in converting the entire healthcare sector from a caring institution to a lucrative industry. Presently Indian healthcare

Table 5.5 Indian Billionaires Whose Wealth Stems from Healthcare or from Pharmaceuticals, 2017[36]

Global Rank	Name	Wealth (Billions US$)	Age	Company	Rank in Indian List
84	Dilip Shanghvi	13.7	61	Sun Pharmaceuticals	4
159	Cyrus Poonawalla	8.1	76	Serum Institute of India	7
303	Pankaj Paid	5.2	64	Cadila Pharmaceuticals	13
34	DeshBandhu Gupta	4.7	79	Lupin Pharmaceuticals	15
501	Ajay Piramal	3.7	62	Piramal	21
660	BR. Shetly	3	75	NMC Healthcare	31
782	P.V. Ramprasad Reddy	2.6	59	Aurobindo Pharma	34=
867	Hasmukh Chudgar	2.4	83	Intas Pharmaceuticals	44=
1030	LeenaTewari	2	59	USV	49
1290	Muruli Divi	1.6	66	Divi's Pharmaceuticals	62=
1376	Yusuf Hamied	1.5	81	Cipla	68=
1567	HabilKhorakiwala	1.3	74	Wockhardt	80=
1567	ShamsheerVayalil	1.3	411	VPS Healthcare	80=
1678	Mahendra Prasad	1.2	77	Aristo Pharmaceuticals	89=
1671	AnaIjit Singh	1.2	63	Max Healthcare	89=
1195	Satish Mehta	1.1	66	Emcure Pharmaceuticals	93=
1795	Samprada Singh	1.1	91	Album Laboratories	93=
1940	Chirayu Amin	1	70	Alembic Pharmaceuticals	97=
1940	Azad Moopen	1	64	Aster DM Healthcare	97=

industry is composed of several interconnected segments. Seventy-seven per cent of it is composed of hospitals, 14 per cent of pharmaceuticals, 6 per cent of medical device sector and 3 per cent of diagnostic services.[37]

However, in a third-world country like India, these changes in the overall healthcare sector widened the gap between the rich and the poor. The 'ability to pay' factor started to play a dominant role in determining the utilization pattern of the health services by the various social classes.

Scenario of West Bengal and Kolkata

As has been pointed out in Chapter 4, the health department in West Bengal from 2006 onwards has recorded the growth of the private healthcare sector separately. In order to understand the growth of the private (corporate) healthcare sector in the post-liberalized era, the sources on which we depend are the documents published by the Department of Health and Family Welfare, Government of West Bengal. But there are several ambiguities between what has been recorded in *Health on the March* and the *Directory of Medical Institutions*. The data are not properly updated.

Thus we have depended upon the list under the Clinical Establishment Act where the private healthcare organizations are registered. There are more than 653 private healthcare organizations[38] (including diagnostic centres, pathological laboratories, nursing homes and private hospitals) in Kolkata. Among these, there are 352 investigation centres (including MRI, CT Scan, ECG, EEG, USG, etc.), pathological laboratories and X-ray clinics. Thirty-two organizations are registered as having outpatient department (OPD) only. These are mainly doctors' chambers or clinics where an individual practitioner or a group of practitioners practise privately. Almost all the diagnostics centres have ultrasonography (USG) facilities and 77 of them have an OPD attached.

In the list of private healthcare organizations, registered under the Clinical Establishments Act, there are 240 nursing homes and private hospitals. Of these, 25 (10.42 per cent) are small nursing homes having one to four beds. There are 62 (25.83 per cent) nursing homes which have five to nine beds each. The number of nursing homes having 10–19 beds is 77 (32.08 per cent). Moreover, there are 56 (23.33 per cent) nursing homes and private hospitals in Kolkata having 20–49 beds. Interestingly, there are only nine (3.75 per cent) private hospitals with beds numbering between 50 and 99. The number of hospitals having more than 100 beds is only 11 (4.58 per cent). The figures are given in a tabular form below (see Table 5.6).

Small nursing homes, where the bed strength is not above ten, have only inpatient care and occasionally an attached OPD. Often, along with the increase in the number of beds in a particular nursing home or hospital, additional services and facilities (investigation, ambulance, canteen, etc.) also become available.

Under the West Bengal Clinical Establishments Act of 1950, it is mandatory for all nursing homes to get registered. However, the list of registered nursing homes available with the state health department does not show their date of establishment. Instead, it shows the date of renewal of the registration. As a result, it is difficult to have an idea of the growth of private nursing homes over the years. There is also the absence of crucial information on a large number of establishments.

There is no doubt though that the private healthcare sector in Kolkata is huge, varied, complex and heterogeneous in character. Any uniform or singular pattern of growth cannot be identified. Over the years this sector has expanded, diversified and become one of the significant healthcare providers in the country (see Table 5.7).

The total number of hospital beds in the private healthcare sector in Kolkata that could be clearly accounted for is 4,247. Out of these, 92 (1.7 per cent) beds are in the nursing homes having bed strength ranging from one to four. A total of 214 (3.96 per cent) beds are available in the nursing homes having bed strength

Table 5.6 Private Nursing Homes and Hospitals – Bed Strength Distribution

Bed Strength	Number	Percentage of the Whole
1–4	25	10.42
5–9	62	25.83
10–19	77	32.08
20–49	56	23.33
50–99	9	3.75
>99	11	4.58
All	**240**	**100**

Table 5.7 Private Healthcare Institutions in Kolkata Registered under the Clinical Establishments Act

Organizations	Number	Percentage (%)
Investigation Centres (Pathology, Radiology, Scan, MRI)	339	51.9
Private Nursing Homes and Hospitals	240	36.75
Day Care Centres (DCC)	17	2.64
Collection Centres	8	1.23
Outpatient Departments	32	4.9
Organizations about which There Is Inadequate Information	17	2.6
All	653	100

Table 5.8 Number of Beds in Establishments of Different Sizes

Nursing Homes with Bed Strength	Beds	Percentage of Beds to Total Number of Beds
1–4	92	2.17
5–9	214	5.04
10–19	590	13.89
20–49	1,123	26.44
50–99	571	13.44
>99	1,601	37.70
Total for 17 daycare centres	56	1.32
All	4,247	100

between 5 and 9. Nursing homes having bed strength between 10 and 19 have 590 (10.93 per cent) beds altogether. A total of 1,123 (20.80 per cent) beds are in nursing homes having bed strength ranging from 20 to 49. On the other hand, 571 (10.58 per cent) and 1,601 (29.65 per cent) beds are in the nursing homes and private hospitals having a number of beds ranging from 50 to 99 and above 100 respectively. Seventeen daycare centres have 56 (1.04 per cent) beds in total (see Table 5.8).

From the above description, it is clear that most of the beds are available in larger private establishments. More than 51 per cent of the beds belong to the two largest categories and almost 78 per cent of the beds belong to the three largest categories. Since the larger categories include the famed multi-speciality establishments that are the most expensive, it goes without saying that a large chunk of the beds in the private sector is out of reach for the common people.

However on the other hand, following *Health on the March (2016–2018)* and *Directory of Medical Institutions (2018)*, there are 401 private hospitals/nursing homes of varied sizes in Kolkata. Out of which nearly 40 have bed strength above 100 and they fall in the tertiary sector. Twenty-nine hospitals/nursing homes have bed strength ranging from 50 to 100. Nearly 150 nursing homes have bed strength between 10 to 50 and the rest have bed strength below 10. But mention should be made as the data is not updated, most of the nursing homes with low bed strength have completely shut down their services (discussed in Chapter 3) but their presence in the *Directory* list is recorded. This faulty approach on behalf of the government creates ambiguities and confusion. Further, it also prevents us from having a concrete scenario of the private healthcare sector in post-liberalized Kolkata quantitatively.

In the case of India, as we have seen there is the significant presence of the corporate sector in healthcare, the same condition prevailed in Kolkata. Apart from corporate companies like Apollo and Fortis, there were several other companies which established hospitals in Kolkata as well as in West Bengal.[39] Narayana Hrudalaya, a Bangalore-based hospital group established many hospitals in Kolkata. Bengal Faith Healthcare Pvt Ltd in 2006 announced the setting up of Bardhaman Health City Project at Bardhaman, West Bengal, at a capital outlay of Rs 1,000 crore. Global Sunrise MediServices Pvt Ltd announced a Multi Organ Transplant Hospital Project Phase I in October 2004 at Rajarhat North 24 Parganas, Bengal at a capital outlay of Rs 150 crores. B.P. Poddar Hospital & Medical Research Pvt announced in 2007 an extension of its Kolkata Hospital in Kolkata from 123 to 260 beds. Himadri Memorial Cancer Welfare Trust was setting up a 150-bed cancer hospital in Kolkata at a cost of Rs 25 crore. Ruby General Hospital Ltd, set up by an NRI doctor, announced the expansion of its Kolkata Hospital to 300 beds at a cost of Rs 10 crore. Beginning its journey with Medica North Bengal Clinic (MNBC) in Siliguri in 2008, the Group launched its flagship Hospital – Medica Superspecialty Hospital (MSH) – in Kolkata in 2010 soon after Medica Cancer Hospital in Rangapani, Siliguri, fulfilled the dire need of a comprehensive cancer facility in North Bengal, and the trust hospital R.C. Agarwal Memorial run by Medica in Tinsukia brought quality multispecialty healthcare to Assam. B.M. Birla Heart Research Centre announced in 2008 the setting up of three hospitals in Rajarhat, 24-Parganas; Siliguri, Darjeeling and Haldia; these are all in West Bengal. The M.P. Birla Group ran a 150-bed hospital and a 46-bed ophthalmology hospital in Kolkata. The Group was planning to set up another budget hospital of nearly 200 beds in Kolkata. The Todi Group (Emami) took over the Niramoy Polyclinic (a government polyclinic) and established the AMRI hospital in Kolkata in 1996. Peerless group also founded a private hospital in the eastern fringes of Kolkata in 1995. Goenkas, Birlas and Kotharis, all have invested on healthcare and established private hospitals in Kolkata. Along with Kolkata, districts also have shown significant presence of the private healthcare sector in various forms. The table below will show the number of private hospitals and hospital beds in West Bengal (see Table 5.9).

From Table 5.9 we can also infer that the growth of the private healthcare sector is not only confined to Kolkata. Almost all the districts have exhibited sharp growth in the rise of private hospitals and nursing homes. The districts of Haora, Hooghly, North and South 24-Parganas, Pashchim Medinipur, Purba Medinipur, Murshidabad, Purulia and Purba Bardhaman have a substantial presence of private hospitals. In these districts and also in other districts of West Bengal, the private

Table 5.9 Medical Institutions and the Number of Sanctioned Beds in the District of West Bengal[40]

District / Health District	Department of Health & Family Welfare Government of West Bengal																	Hospital under Other Departments of State Government***		Local Bodies		Government of India 1		NGO Private 1		Total	
	Medical College Hospital		District Hospital		Sub-Divisional Hospital		State General Hospital		Other Hospital*		Rural Hospital		Block Primary Health Centre		Primary Health Centre**											
	No.	Total No. of Beds	No.	Total No. of Beds	No.	Total No. of Beds	No.	Total No. of Beds	No.	Total No. of Beds	No.	Total No. of Beds	No.	Total No. of Beds	No.	Total No. of Beds	No.	Total No. of Beds	No.	Total No. of Beds	No.	Total No. of Beds	No.	Total No. of Beds	No.	Total No. of Beds
Alipurduar	0	0	1	370	0	0	1	220	0	0	7	210	0	0	13	98	1	9	0	0	2	161	18	453	43	1521
Bankura	1	1441	0	0	1	114	0	0	1	550	14	480	2	45	40	352	2	25	0	0	2	28	32	705	131	4435
131B4465ishmupur HD	0	0	1	300	0	0	0	0	0	0	5	190	1	20	23	162										
PurbaBarddhaman	1	1211	0	0	2	484	0	0	0	0	15	530	10	210	74	533	2	79	0	0	1	5	102	2719	207	5771
Paschim Barddhaman	0	0	1	450	1	282	0	0	0	0	7	230	2	40	32	209	2	170	0	0	17	2819	57	2390	119	6590
Birbhum	0	0	1	342	1	224	0	0	1	300	9	300	2	75	36	290	3	14	0	0	3	50	50	1004	137	3579
Rampurhat HD	1	326	0	0	0	0	0	0	0	0	6	200	2	60	23	194										
Dakshin Dinajpur	0	0	0	432	1	300	0	0	0	0	6	250	2	10	18	180	1	50	1	25	0	0	14	255	44	1502
Darjeeling	2	599	2	595	1	120	0	0	3	384	7	260	2	40	16	124	5	91	1	24	6	475	60	2421	104	5403
Haora	0	0	1	542	1	589	6	653	1	52	13	548	2	30	43	435	6	996	0	0	0	101	172	3246	246	7250
Hugli	0	0	1	650	3	814	0	204	1	55	17	630	1	10	60	462	7	817	2	193	1	4	264	3676	358	7515
Jalpaiguri	0	0	1	700	0	100	0	0	1	60	6	250	1	10	26	176	2	46	0	0	2	200	24	646	54	2188
Kalimpong	0	0	1	370	0	0	0	0	0	0	2	60	1	25	5	48	2	28	0	0	0	0	7	127	19	858
Koch Bihar	1	500	0	0	4	570	0	0	2	150	8	240	4	60	29	228	2	40	0	0	1	2	21	634	72	2544
Kolkata	5	8129	0	0	0	0	0	0	21	4821	0	0	0	0	0	0	9	1711	6	305	8	3072	400	16757	449	34798
Malda	1	1000	0	0	0	100	0	0	1	30	16	515	0	0	34	270	2	40	1	15	1	100	36	838	93	2908
Murshidabad	1	1157	0	0	4	1062	0	0	1	350	17	580	10	205	70	574	5	223	2	70	1	3	118	2360	229	6584

(Continued)

Table 5.9 (Continued)

District / Health District	Department of Health & Family Welfare Government of West Bengal																		Local Bodies		Government of India 1		NGO Private 1		Total	
	Medical College Hospital		District Hospital		Sub-Divisional Hospital		State General Hospital		Other Hospital*		Rural Hospital		Block Primary Health Centre		Primary Health Centre**		Hospital under Other Departments of State Government***									
	No.	Total No. of Beds	No.	Total No. of Beds	No.	Total No. of Beds	No.	Total No. of Beds	No.	Total No. of Beds	No.	Total No. of Beds	No.	Total No. of Beds	No.	Total No. of Beds	No.	Total No. of Beds	No.	Total No. of Beds	No.	Total No. of Beds	No.	Total No. of Beds	No.	Total No. of Beds
Nadia	1	900	1	700	2	350	3	356	4	2305	14	460	3	30	47	404	3	345	0	0	1	10	90	1538	189	7688
North 24 Parganas	1	500	1	600	3	652	7	711	0	0	9	270	3	45	28	210	6	603	11	356	3	272	160	5606	266	10915
Basirhat HD	0	0	1	300	0	0	0	0	0	0	9	370	1	15	23	206	0	0	1	10	3		127			
Paschim Medinipur	1	771	0	0	2	556	0	0	2	351	17	695	4	95	58	414	4	319	1	10	3	446	127	1487	219	5114
Jhargram	0	0	1	300	0	0	0	0	0	0	8	300		0	25	200	0	0	0	0	0		10	115	44	915
Purba Medinipur	0	0	1	500	2	450	1	50	0	0	10	300	5	75	29	220	0	0	0	0	1	47			242	5133
Nandigram HD	0	0	1	180	1	206	0	0	0	0	5	150	4	85	22	189	0	0	0	0	1		160	2681		
Puruliya	1	537	0	0	1	200	0	0	1	190	18	620	2	40	54	383	2	43	0	0	2	206	23	665	104	2896
South 24-Parganas	0	0	2	625	2	218	4	524	0	0	12	370	5	65	31	242	0	0	5	80	1	143	153	2839	214	5136
Diamond Harbour HD	1	332	0	0	1	100	0	0	0	0	9	360	4	100	29	236	0	0	0	0	1		44		44	1128
Uttar Dinajpur	1	400	0	0	1	249	1	60	0	0	6	180	3	60	19	132	1	50	0	0	0	0	21	330	53	1461
Total	18	17803	18	8626	36	7840	24	2778	40	9598	273	9546	75	1470	913	7191	67	5672	30	1083	57	8146	2139	53892	3890	133845

Total Number of Sanctioned Beds in SNCU, SNSU, CCU, HOU, PICU, MCH Hubs — 6385

Total Sanctioned Beds in Multi / Super Specialty Hospitals — 13800

Total Beds — 153804

healthcare was chiefly identified with secondary care hospitals which are actually small nursing homes with very limited infrastructure. Tertiary care however was mostly absent in the districts.

The Reforms or 'Dictates': Impact of Liberalization in Public Hospitals in West Bengal

The World Bank's proposal to reduce the role of the public health services and to promote the growth of the private healthcare sector brought about a catastrophe in the entire healthcare services of the country.

The World Development Report 1993 (WDR)[41] stated that both the public and private sectors had important roles in the delivery of healthcare services, but the state-funded health system in many developing countries needed to be restructured and reformed. The changes could be made through legal and administrative means designed to facilitate private (NGO and for-profit) involvement in the provision of health services, by public subsidies to NGOs for supplying the essential package and by curtailment of new investments in public tertiary hospitals.[42]

The World Bank gave a total amount of US$350 million as loan over 35 years, repayable at 12 per cent per annum. This loan was initially given to four states that were selected out of the ten states which submitted proposals for reforming their healthcare sector under the State Health System Projects. Four states were selected for undertaking the reforms based on heterogeneity of the country in terms of epidemiological profiles, levels of economic development, health services development and political structures.

The impact of the reforms in India did exhibit a miserable state of affairs. A number of scholars have documented a series of changes, which the reforms brought about in the healthcare sector.[43]

The Government of West Bengal published a document titled 'Public Private Partnership' (PPP) on 6 October 2004 in its official website www.wbhealth.gov .in boldly announcing its intention to privatize the government health sector systematically. It set up the target of attracting 80 per cent of the total health budget as investment from private business houses in the next ten years. However, the preparation for this paradigm shift started back in November 1992 when it introduced fees for outdoor tickets in government hospitals, levied charges for diagnostic investigation, reduced the number of free beds, etc. This was done to show allegiance to the conditions laid down by the World Bank for its loan of Rs 701 crore which started coming in 1995. In accordance with the second phase of structural adjustment for which Department for International Development (DFID), UK provided a loan of Rs 745 crore, the user fees were increased and free services became more and more restricted. The supply of free medicines and other appliances was also constricted.[44] (However, presently, user fees are not charged in government hospitals in West Bengal. This will be discussed in the segment 'New Strategies: Some Steps forward').

On 1 August 1995, the then health minister of West Bengal, Prasanta Sur, announced that the state government had taken a loan of Rs 600 crore from the

World Bank. The Left Front government in West Bengal did not have any hesitation to accept the conditionalities imposed by the Bank.[45]

On the other hand, the 17th report of the Assembly Standing Committee on Health[46] observed that India's attempt to develop self-sufficiency in healthcare delivery in the 1960s and 1970s was reversed in the late 1980s and 1990s by the Union government. It said that the change in scenario was a reflection of the changes in international politics. The multinationals were operating through projects aided by the IMF, World Bank and various other external agencies. These were becoming dominant in recent years. According to the committee, these projects were 'unifactoral' and did not commensurate with the needs of the common people. In practice, it was creating more dependence on the diagnostic and therapeutic measures only. Healthcare delivery based on the universalization of social justice had been put in the cold storage.[47]

The Left Front parties, by virtue of their politics, generally took a negative attitude towards the World Bank loans. However, as a representative of the state, the minister of the department concerned gladly expressed willingness of the government for initiating reforms in public healthcare sector under projects funded by the Bank. Nevertheless, in 1988, chief minister Jyoti Basu had also admitted the failure of the public healthcare infrastructure and invited private entrepreneurs for providing healthcare.

The World Bank provided Rs 701 crore for The State Health Sector Development Project (SHSDP) – II, aimed at improving 170 secondary-level hospitals and 36 primary health centres in the Sunderbans. Civil work was done with World Bank assistance in a number of state hospitals in the late 1990s. Funds were also provided to purchase medicines and equipments. Apart from this, considerable progress was made in hospital waste management, disease surveillance, quality assurance and training of health personnel. The nurse–doctor ratio steadily improved in the state. In 1997 it was 1:10, compared to 1:18 in the previous year.[48]

The state government was exploring various ways of improving the quality of service from medical facilities under its control. In a move to involve the beneficiaries in the running of primary health centres, it decided to hand over some of the primary health centres to the panchayat bodies and NGOs.[49]

Vacant posts of teachers under the West Bengal Medical Education Service were filled up through walk-in interviews in a very short period of time. Hysteroscopes, ultrasonograph machines and laparoscope instruments for different abdominal operations were installed in different medical colleges for better teaching and research and patient care. At R.G. Kar Medical College, a new intensive treatment unit was opened. The ICCU in the department of cardiology at this hospital was restructured and renovated. The emergency ward at Calcutta National Medical College was also renovated. A magnetic resonance imaging (MRI) instrument was installed at the Bangur Institute of Neurology. An operation theatre and casualty block with observation beds were constructed in Bankura Sammilani Medical College. A dialysis unit was opened at Sambhunath Pandit Hospital. The heritage building of Calcutta Medical College was renovated.

In order to assist in the management of hospitals, the state government developed a Health Management Information System (HMIS). Under HMIS, a standardized recording, reporting and feedback system was to be developed for all the hospitals. HMIS was fully implemented in the district and sub-divisional hospitals, as well as state general hospitals with 200-plus beds.

Indo-German Basic Health Project[50]

GTZ-KFW funded Basic Health Project (BHP) was initiated in 2001 in eight districts of the state. In the first phase, civil work for the rehabilitation of 38 BPHCs and 92 PHCs and the construction of 95 sub-centres were taken up in these districts. Rehabilitation of 75 BPHCs and 30 PHCs was taken up in the second phase during 2005–2006. Ambulance services at the basic healthcare level were also introduced.[51]

European Commission Assisted Sector Investment Programme[52]

The European Commission sanctioned a grant of Rs 45.2 crore under the Sector Investment Programme, which started in February 2002. The Government of India released the funds directly to the West Bengal State Health and Family Welfare Department. The activities included:

- Organizational Restructuring.
- Integration of management of externally assisted programmes and projects.
- Derivation of Hospital Reports through Management Information System.
- Capacity building of district Family Welfare Samitis.

Apart from these, assistance was given to some other programmes. These were:[53]

- Urban Health Improvement Plan in six municipalities within KMDA area.
- School health programme.
- State Thalassemia Control Programme.
- Strengthening of Health Management Information System and introduction of e-management in the health system in the districts.

DFID-Assisted Health Sector Development Initiative[54]

DFID and West Bengal State Health and Family Welfare Samiti signed an agreement in August 2005 for the former's support to strategic planning and sector reform cell of the department of health and family welfare. The World Bank also proposed to collaborate with the Government of West Bengal in its initiative for improving the primary healthcare system. A joint appraisal mission of the DFID and World Bank visited the state during March 7–17, 2005, for finalizing the project.[55]

From the above discussion, it seems that the health sector reforms in West Bengal under the SHSDP II had brought certain glaring improvements in the overall healthcare infrastructure. However, there is another side of the story. The blueprint of public–private partnership (PPP) was promoted from this time onwards. Although official documents have emphasized the positive impact of the health sector reforms, these reforms deepened the crisis by transforming healthcare into a marketable commodity. In accordance with the second phase of structural adjustment for which DFID provided a loan of Rs 745 crore, the user fees increased and free services became more and more restricted. The supply of free medicines and other appliances was also constricted.[56]

The state has also identified private nursing homes as one of the important healthcare delivery sectors in its official documents. Yet, 90 per cent of the hospitalization cases in the rural areas and 71 per cent in the urban areas continued to take place in the public hospitals. It should be taken into account that the high rate of utilization of the public healthcare services and admission in public hospitals in no way represent the trust of the majority of the people in public healthcare. The percentage of patients being completely cured by utilizing these facilities should be the real indicator of the performance of the public hospitals. Installing high-tech medical equipment in the public hospitals also did not necessarily increase the efficiency of these units. These were bought at a high cost from multinational companies and often lay unused or went out of order due to lack of maintenance. Moreover, political pressure crippled the health sector administration.

The next phase of privatization witnessed the transferring of government hospitals to private investors in the name of PPP. For example, a specialized TB hospital at Jadavpur, Kolkata, having 750 indoor beds in a sprawling area of 200 *bighas*, was leased to a private group for just Re 1 to set up a private medical college. Incidentally, it was the first private medical college in West Bengal and soon gained a reputation for underhand dealing, capitation fees and other irregularities in admission of students along with doubtful teaching standards.[57]

We will take a deeper look into the privatization of the K.S. Roy TB Hospital. It was established in 1938. Since in India a large number of people were affected by tuberculosis, the need was felt for a separate place for treating TB patients with specialized care (including isolation, open space for fresh air and long-term stay in the hospital having proper cross-ventilation facilities) and the K.S. Roy TB Hospital provided all these.

But, the state health department had made several attempts to sell this hospital since the 1980s. A 'TB Haspatal bachao Committee' (Committee to Save TB Hospital) was set up by the local people to protest against the government's move. Finally, in 2004, the entire property was leased to KPC group for Re 1.

Kali Prasad Chaudhuri (KPC), a US-based NRI orthopaedic surgeon, was the sponsor of the private medical college and hospital which came upon the premises. Since his declared aim was to 'serve the community with health care facilities at reasonable prices,' the outdoor ticket was made available at Rs 10. The abnormally low cost of treatment in the outdoor section of the private hospital was widely advertised in many parts of the city. Soon the user charges were increased to Rs 50 and in many cases even to Rs 150. Like many other private hospitals, there were many allegations of inflated bills and in some instances, the patients were shifted to other places being unable to cope with the high charges.[58]

Three more hospitals at Kamarhati, Dhubulia and Dubrajpur were also up for sale. The hospital at Kamarhati was all set to be handed over to Apollo Gleneagles when a protest by the local residents and workers of a political party stalled it.

Low-paid contractual staff was replacing regular staff in all spheres, important programme components and non-clinical support services were being assigned to NGOs and all district-level health activities were transferred to the District Health and Family Welfare Samity, controlled by the Zila Parishad Sabadhipati, DM (District Magistrate) and representative of the local MP (Member of Parliament), among others. In a survey conducted in 2007, it was seen that among the 922 health centres of West Bengal, 111 did not have any doctor, 257 had no lab-technician and 66 centres had no pharmacist. Amongst the nursing staff, several posts were vacant and 2,486 new posts were required to be created.[59]

Overall, though a huge extra-budgetary transaction was noted, the State Health System Development Project II intended to develop middle-tier hospitals (rural to district hospitals) and a proper patient referral system turned out to be a flop. The common people failed to achieve any benefit from this project due to lack of proper planning, fragmented approach, lack of coordination among various departments, reluctance on the part of service providers, etc. On the other hand, a group of corrupt party leaders, corrupt administrators, contractors, a section of doctors and health staff siphoned off the funds.[60]

The impact of SHSDP on primary healthcare further provided the space for privatization of this sector. According to the national norm, one PHC should cater to a population of 30,000 in a rural area. In the case of hilly and tribal areas, one PHC should serve around 20,000 people. Moreover, according to government rule, there will be at least two doctors (MBBS) in the OPD and a basic infrastructure for treating general diseases. In complicated cases where the patient needs admission for long-term treatment, he or she is referred to a secondary-level hospital (sub-divisional, district, state general or special hospital). But in reality, due to lack of infrastructure in the PHCs, even patients suffering from general diseases are referred to secondary hospitals which do not have the infrastructure to handle the load. As a result, the entire referral systems collapse and the rural masses are either shifted to the unqualified quacks of the villages or to small nursing homes which are becoming increasingly popular.

According to the 2001 census, the district of Hooghly in West Bengal has a population of 33,34,227. It should have 112 PHCs. But this district has nine-block primary health centres (BPHCs) and 61 PHCs. Another 42 PHCs are needed to fulfil the requirement. Moreover, in most of the PHCs, there is only one doctor who treats 50–100 patients within 2–3 hours daily. This indicates that a patient gets less than two minutes' attention from a doctor.

The SHSDP proposed to convert BPHCs to 'Rural Hospitals' where along with high-tech, imported equipments, there would be one anaesthetist, one gynaecologist, one paediatrician and one radiologist. The World Bank forced the government to purchase the instruments from the multinational companies (selected by the Bank) but refused to finance the salary of the medical personnel. Moreover, there was a dearth of these specialists required for the rural hospitals in the West Bengal Health Service. As a result, the government failed to provide adequate manpower in the rural hospitals. As an alternative option, it was decided to recruit doctors on contract. However, this also did not bring about any solution to the problem because these categories of specialists are in limited number. So why will they opt for contractual jobs? Thus, the World Bank-funded projects silently ruined the entire primary healthcare infrastructure in the name of reforms. The World Bank skillfully concentrated its reforms in such places which will be advantageous for its profit. More than 30 per cent of the medical equipments remained unused in most rural hospitals.

As far as the development of primary-level public infrastructure for health is concerned, the West Bengal government was categorical about consolidating and upgrading existing infrastructure rather than proliferating ill-equipped infrastructure. It did not want to add new PHCs, which are the first referral points for rural areas where doctors and some rudimentary medical services are made available. This logic conveniently bypasses and ignores questions as to why, in the first place, infrastructure was not set up in all these years, and why did they remain ill-equipped and dysfunctional.[61]

New Strategies: Some Steps Forward

The present government in West Bengal has undertaken certain long-term measures to reform and restructure the decaying state of public healthcare system. Some of the measures are as follows:[62]

- In an unprecedented move in early 2013, the Government of West Bengal decided to implement a Universal Free Treatment Policy in all state-run hospitals, to reduce the out-of-pocket expenditure of the patients, irrespective of their income level. This included the cost of medicines, consumables, implants, diagnostic expenses, bed charges and all other incidental expenditure that were hitherto borne by the patients.
- Over 28,000 beds have been added to the existing and new government hospitals – enhancing the total number of beds to 83,991.
- 42 Multi/Super Specialty Hospitals with 300/500-bedded facilities each are coming up at a project cost of about Rs 2,714 crore and are opened in several districts of West Bengal.
- 115 Fair Price Medicine Shops are functional, providing discounts ranging from 48 per cent to 77.2 per cent on MRP. Till 31 December 2017, a discount of more than Rs. 1,100 crore had been availed by almost 4 crore people.
- 88 units (12 CT scans, 5 MRI, 38 Digital X-rays and 33 dialysis) are already functional under Public–Private Partnership (PPP) mode.
- Four new 'health districts' at Alipurduar, Kalimpong, Jhargram and Paschim Bardhaman together with five new 'health districts' at Nandigram, Bishnupur,

Rampurhat, Diamond Harbour and Basirhat have taken the number of 'health districts' from 19 to 28. This has helped to streamline and improve the functioning of district-level health administration.

- With a view to augment the availability of nurses, the nursing training schools have increased from 25 in 2011 to 39 in 2018 with a rise in seat capacity from 850 (2011) to 2,175 (2018). One more nursing college has been added taking the number from nine to ten. The seating capacity has also increased from 330 to 860.

- More than 45 lakh families belonging to members of Self Help Groups, ICDS Workers, ASHA Workers, Civic Volunteers Force, Civil Defence Volunteers, selected contractual employees, cable TV operators, etc., have already been enrolled in the 'Swasthya Sathi' health card scheme. In December 2021, it was expanded to cover the state's entire population. The scheme, which was initially launched in 2016, is a basic health cover for secondary and tertiary care up to Rs 5 lakh per annum per family.

- More than 63 lakh families are covered under Rashtriya Swasthya Bima Yojana (RSBY). The number of hospitals empanelled under RSBY has also increased to 1,308 from 1,293 hospitals last year.

- 307 Sick Newborn Stabilisation Unit (SNSU) has been made operational to provide comprehensive neonatal care. No SNSU existed in any government health facility before 2011.

- 68 SNCUs are functional in the State with additional 2,217 beds for providing specialized care to newborns. These have helped significantly to reduce neonatal and infant mortality. Two more SNCUs at Contai SDH and Srerampore SSH became functional from the end of 2017. Only six SNCUs existed before 2011.

- A comprehensive upgradation of infrastructure for maternal, newborn and paediatric services has been undertaken at a cost of Rs 132 crore, which includes the upgradation of labour rooms, labour OTs, maternity wards, neonatal wards, paediatric wards and other service support areas up to PHCs, BPHCs, SGHs and SDHs. A total of 302 labour rooms, 389 OTs, 1,075 toilet blocks and 975 drinking water facilities are being set up as part of this project. In addition, upgradation of 68 hospitals with a delivery load of more than 3,000 per annum are being upgraded, out of which 38 have been upgraded and the rest are under progress.

- With an objective to provide access to Comprehensive Primary Health Care Services including non-communicable diseases like hypertension, diabetes, etc. and other such ailments, it has been planned to upgrade all 10,357 Sub-Centres to Health and Wellness Centres over a period of five years. These will be manned by a Community Health Officer, an in-service GNM Nurse with at least two years' experience after having undergone a six- month bridge course in Community Health, ANMs, Multi-Purpose Workers and ASHA Workers. A projected Rs. 1,000 crore will be invested for this purpose with an annual recurring expenditure of Rs. 800 crore. Presently West Bengal has 5,146 functional health and wellness centres.

- Four government medical colleges (Malda Medical College, College of Medicine and Sagore Dutta Hospital, North 24-Parganas, Murshidabad Medical College, Berhampore and College of Medicine and JNM Hospital, Nadia) and three private medical colleges (IQ City Durgapur, I Care Medical College Haldia, Gouri Devi Institute of Medical Sciences, Durgapur) have been made functional since 2011. Eleven new medical colleges are coming up at Rampurhat (Birbhum), Cooch Behar, Uluberia (Howrah), Arambagh (Hooghly), Jalpaiguri, Jhargram, Barasat (North 24-Parganas), Tamluk (Purba Medinipur), Purulia, Diamond Harbour (South 24-Parganas) and Raigunj (Uttar Dinajpur). An All India Institute of Medical Sciences is coming up at Kalyani. The proposed new Medical Colleges will lead to an addition of almost 1,200 MBBS seats. Out of 11 medical colleges, five (Rampurhat, Cooch Behar, Diamond Harbour, Purulia and Raugunje) are functional since 2018.
- Total 1,345 MBBS and BDS (Dental) seats have been increased in the last seven years, with 100 more in the offing.
- 493 postgraduate seats and 64 post-doctoral seats have been added to the existing medical colleges.
- The government established the West Bengal Health Recruitment Board on 13 September 2012 to expedite the process of recruitment of doctors and other staff under the control of the Department of Health and Family Welfare. More than 27,000 posts of different categories have been created during the last seven years. A total number of 9,770 medical officers have been recruited and permanently engaged. In addition, more than 17,000 nurses, pharmacists and technicians have also been recruited in the last seven years. Additionally, 9,382 posts have been notified to HRB for recruitment. As per the Health Department sources 4,544 doctors, 6,535 nurses, 833 pharmacists and 1,001 technicians have been added to the existing medical and paramedical force of the state. The government in July 2021 had sanctioned the creation of 1,464 new posts of different categories for proposed medical colleges with an intake capacity of 100 MBBS seats each. Those posts included 36 professors, 120 associate professors, 156 assistant professors and 240 RMOs. The six proposed medical colleges will have a total intake capacity of 600 MBBS seats. With a view to retain existing Medical Officers, the age of superannuation for West Bengal Health Services, West Bengal Public Health-cum-Administrative Services and West Bengal Medical Education Services has been raised from 62 years to 65 years.
- 41 Critical Care Units (CCU) and 24 High Dependency Units (HDU) are already functional in tertiary and secondary-level hospitals. No CCU existed in any district or sub-divisional hospitals before 2011. Eleven Paediatric Intensive Care Units are also functional. Four started functioning from 2017.
- 15 Neonatal Intensive Care Units with state-of-the-art ventilation facilities for sick Neonates have been planned in 13 medical colleges including Dr B.C. Roy PGIPS and Chittaranjan Seva Sadan, which are now under different stages of progress.

- The Urban Health Centres started functioning in West Bengal in the financial year 2013–2014 as a subset of the National Health Mission with its goal to address the health concerns of urban population, especially the urban poor. West Bengal Clinical Establishments Regulatory Commission with adequate powers to monitor, supervise and regulate has been constituted with effect from 17 March 2017. The Commission aims to provide quick redressal to the patients aggrieved due to deficiencies in medical services and/or overbilling.
- In coordination with the Municipal Affairs and Urban Development Department, beautification project of the premises of District Hospital, sub-divisional hospital and State General Hospital have been taken up. Beautification has been completed in 16 MCHs and 22 District Hospitals. Work has begun for the beautification of 25 SDHs and SGHs. 5,733 scavengers have been outsourced for scavenging services in all government facilities.
- Decision has been taken to install CCTV cameras for security and surveillance in government hospitals from medical college and hospitals and state general hospitals. This surveillance mechanism has already been installed in 39 of the super speciality/multi-speciality hospitals.

The above-mentioned measures are undoubtedly a leap forward for better public healthcare in West Bengal. But increasing the number of hospitals and hospital beds and that too in the tertiary sector is not a panacea to the growing demand of the huge population living in the interiors of rural Bengal. This is highly evident from the per bed population ratio in rural Bengal which is 1:3,415.[63]

Moreover, as the government has paid more attention to developing the tertiary health sector, rural healthcare is utterly neglected (discussed in Chapter 4) compared to the population. It is interesting to point out that in recent years fashioning of the state-run hospitals as corporate hospitals with decorated waiting lounges, vitrified floorings, airconditioned rooms and 'state of the art technologies' might suggest that radical changes have been brought forward. Giant structures are being constructed with over emphasis on beautification, but the services are still inadequate. In the teaching hospitals, there is acute staff shortage which increases the pressure on the existing system. If the primary healthcare sector had been substantially improved, with very basic requirements for the rural patients, pressure on the 'multispeciality/superspeciality' hospitals would have been lessened. The overcrowding of patients from the districts of West Bengal to the OPDs of medical colleges in Kolkata for the treatment of certain basic ailments (especially communicable diseases) reflects the fact that the rudimentary infrastructure is actually unavailable in the primary health centres and rural hospitals. Rural Health Statistics (2017–2018) show that theoretically out of 908 primary health centres in West Bengal, only 640 are functioning. In rural hospitals there is a dearth of specialists like gynaecologists, surgeons, etc. Ambulances are not available on time to shift the patients to sub-divisional hospitals. By installing high-end instruments in multi-speciality/super speciality hospitals, the state has shifted its focus to treating communicable diseases which require specialized treatments inviting a techno-centric approach in healthcare.

Moreover, by introducing Swasthya Sathi, the government is actually strengthening the intrusion of the private insurance companies in the health sector. Though the allocation of funds has increased from Rs 2,400 crore in 2017–2018 to Rs 6,400 crore in 2019–2020 for Swasthya Sathi/Pradhan Mantri Jan Arogya Yojana, substantial improvements were not visible in National Health Mission or in developing primary healthcare. In November 2020, the West Bengal chief minister announced coverage of the entire population of the state under the insurance of Swasthya Sathi. This increased the allocation from Rs 925 crore to Rs 2,000 crore. In reality, much of the money allocated will move to the private insurance companies, thus once again corporatizing healthcare in a different style.

Problems of the Private/Corporate Healthcare Sector

Corruption, Malpractice and Negligence: Issues of Medical Ethics

Healthcare services are characterized by certain well-known peculiarities and inherent market failures: asymmetric information, adverse selection, moral hazard, uncertainity on numerous dimension, externalities and so on. All of the features provide strong arguments for government across the world to regulate the provision of healthcare. Historically the Indian government has been mandated to play all three roles, that is, provider, financer and regulator. But in a privatized healthcare system that exists in a country like India, the role of the state has been minimised.[64]

The consequences of a private sector-led model of provisioning are well known – distortions, induced consumptions, a drive towards more technology-intensive care and, above all, high cost of care. One of the reasons why the private sector needs to indulge in such unethical practices is the failure to achieve economies of scale for the investments made in capital-intensive equipment and diagnostics. In order to create product discrimination and provide 'state of the art' technologies, there is always a tendency to over supply some of the high-end services like computer tomography (CT) scans, magnetic resonance imaging (MRI), etc. It is often the case that if one follows standard treatment protocols, given the patient load, usage would be less and hence returns would be less compared to investments made to procure such services. Consequences of private sector-led growth on people are well-documented. Evidence of RSBY suggests that cashless insurance mechanisms fail to reduce out-of-pocket expenditure. Insurance schemes are always for inpatient treatment. The same mechanisms would prevail under managed care model and there is no reason to believe that exploitation of the poor would stop. Global experience suggests that most developing countries do not have the capacity to regulate the private health sector and especially corporate hospitals. In India, there is very limited experience in terms of regulating the private sector. Until recently there were no efforts to enumerate the total private health enterprises at the national level. Thus, the question of regulation has been limited to the field of manufacturing, sale, quality and prescription of drugs and pharmaceuticals medical and clinical practice related to registration and inspection of facilities. Apart from these, there are legislations in some states for registering the private sector. Though these legislations exist on paper, there is hardly any initiative from the state governments to even register private clinical establishments.[65] This is also true in the case of West Bengal.

In a corporatized atmosphere where healthcare is a commodity, the hospitals with their five-star hospitality services have changed the notion of what a hospital can or should be. Hospitals are no longer places for providing the health services that are needed for patients in a comfortable setting but have become sites for fulfilling desires of hospitality services in a luxurious ambience.[66]

Prescribing costly drugs and sometimes unnecessary investigations, the branded 'healthcare malls' are selling their wide range of products to the patients who are further sickened by the interventionist role of medicines. The more a patient is confined within the four walls of the hospital, the more profit is reaped by the healthcare industry. The medicalized atmosphere of the hospital does not cure patients holistically. It tries to retain the sickness around the patient who always suffers from the tendency of getting sick again. Sickness brings money or capital, which violates the ethics of the medical profession. The private healthcare sector is plagued by all these ills associated with the business.

These hospitals have ensured their profits by giving doctors targets to be fulfilled through available patient loads. The doctors become merely workers in such hospitals where they are converted to consultants from specialists. The nature of practice thus changed from that of family doctors to consultants offering services in big hospitals with a consultant-client relationship.[67]

Corruption is not just limited to clinical practice, but extends to policymaking. Here the nature and scale of corrupt practices at the highest levels of health technocracy are different and have implications for larger numbers of both providers and recipients of health services.[68]

Antia has pointed out that the medical profession has enjoyed a uniquely privileged position because of its technical skill as well as the intensely personal relationship which develops between a doctor and his patient. The latter puts his/her entire faith in the doctor who not only cures but also cares and consoles the patient as well as the patient's family. The epithet 'noble' is symbolic of the love and respect that this profession has enjoyed over the years.[69]

Dr N.C. Das, a senior anaesthetist of Kolkata, observes that in earlier times most of the doctors were general practitioners with an MBBS or LMF degree. They used to carry injection syringes and emergency drugs and were able to undertake even minor surgeries. Sending patients to hospitals or nursing homes was not very common in those days. The general physicians or the family physicians who were also close to the family members cured minor health problems at home. They enjoyed a position of love and respect. The emergence of the specialists and consultants, along with the changing disease profile brought about a decline in their social status and public esteem.[70]

The indiscriminate use of the intensive care units even for terminal patients increases the profitability or the salability of the product of the medical institution and results in aggravating the pain of the patient rather than giving him relief. Each techno-centric facility has its specific limited use, but when deliberately pushed to their limit by the 'technical robots' (doctors) for satisfying their monetary greed, the wonders of modern science prove to be counter-productive.[71] The scale of corruption multiplies in the case of unnecessary MRIs, CT scans, hysterectomy, cardiac stents, and bypass surgeries. Ruthless profiteering practices in the healthcare sector have vulnerable and weak patients at the receiving end with inelastic demand for rational medical needs.[72]

The practice of extending the stay at hospital, unnecessary admission in ICU and ascribing disease to make patients out of healthy persons and converting them to lifelong patients became the order of the corporate healthcare culture.[73]

The growing middle class has now been caught in a cleft stick between providing the latest medical care like renal dialysis, kidney transplant and coronary bypass surgery and are pauperized in the bargain. Many search for old-fashioned family doctors who are now reducing in number due to the overwhelming presence of specialists and consultants.[74]

In a privatized healthcare system a patient is converted to a customer or a consumer and the doctor is either a shareholder, proprietor or partner of the hospital. The doctor–patient relationship has become one of extracting the most profit out of the patient. As the 'business' deal becomes the primary mode of interaction, a significant lack of trust is visible in the doctor–patient relation.

Diagonistic set-ups within a hospital and outside the ambit of hospital management give 30 to 50 per cent of the cost of an MRI or a CT scan to the referring doctor. For laboratory tests, the range is 20–30 per cent. This level of kickbacks makes it impossible for many laboratories to maintain their integrity while carrying out all prescribed tests. Many of the tests prescribed by a doctor are only meant to push up the bill and thus his own commission. Hence a lot of the samples collected from apparently healthy looking people are thrown into the sink, and are referred to as the 'sink tests'. This can be dangerous for patients, as genuine ailments sometimes remain undiagnosed.[75]

In a complex high-technology hospital, negligence[76] becomes 'random human error', callousness becomes 'scientific detachment' and incompetence becomes 'lack of specialized equipment'. The depersonalization of diagnosis and therapy has turned malpractices from an ethical into a technical problem[77]

What has been put forward in 'Society and Health: the dilemma'[78] seems more pertinent to the changing scenario of healthcare culture today. The boom in biological sciences in the last three decades has brought with it an emphasis on producing the scientific physician – highly trained, specialized in analyzing data and skilled in the diagnosis and treatment of organic diseases. Medical students are well inculcated with the importance of laboratory and clinical investigation. The students are educated in an atmosphere in which the 'good patient' is the sick patient, who has multiple physical, radiological and laboratory abnormalities.[79]

However, most medical schools focus on two primary goals:

- To provide opportunity to learn the technical and scientific skills required to treat disease.
- To learn the necessary techniques required to understand the social and cultural milieu of the physician-patient relationship

But the adequate emphasis on the second has been lost. By graduation, physicians have to be prepared to take immediate, scientifically based action in treating ill individuals but they are often unable to visualize and understand the social context in which both they and their patients function.[80]

The *Global Corruption Report* has raised the question as to why are health systems are prone to corruption.[81]

Corruption in the health sector is not exclusive to any particular kind of health system. It occurs in systems whether they are predominantly public or private, well funded or poorly funded, technically simple or sophisticated. The extent of corruption is, in part, a reflection of the society in which it operates. Health system corruption is less likely in societies where there is broad adherence to the rule of law, transparency and trust, and where the public sector is ruled by effective civil service codes and strong accountability mechanisms.

These general factors affect the extent of corruption in any sector, but the health sector has a number of dimensions that make it particularly vulnerable to abuse. No other sector has the specific mix of uncertainty, asymmetric information and large number of dispersed actors that characterize the health sector. As a result, susceptibility to corruption is a systemic feature of health systems, and controlling it requires policies that address the sector as a whole.

Two other factors that contribute to corruption in healthcare are worth mentioning. First, the scope of corruption in the health sector may be wider than in other sectors because society frequently entrusts private actors in health with important public roles. When private pharmaceutical companies, hospitals or insurers act dishonestly to enrich themselves, they are not formally abusing 'public office for private gain'. Nevertheless, they are abusing the public's trust in the sense that people and organizations engaged in health service delivery are held to a higher standard in the interests of protecting people's health. The medical profession, in particular, is given great latitude in most countries to police itself in return for assuming professional responsibility to act in the best interest of patients.

Uncertainty is a central feature of the health sector and has far-reaching implications, as was first argued by Kenneth Arrow in 1963.[82] Arrow showed that uncertainty regarding who will fall ill, when illness will occur, what kinds of illnesses people get and how efficacious treatments are, make the market for healthcare services very different from other markets in terms of the scope for market failure. Due to uncertainty, medical care service markets and health insurance markets are both likely to be inefficient.

This uncertainty makes it difficult for those demanding medical care – patients or their families – to discipline suppliers of medical care, as occurs in other markets. Patients cannot shop around for the best price and quality when they are ignorant of the costs, alternatives and precise nature of their needs. In such situations, consumer choices do not reflect price and quality in the normal fashion, and other mechanisms – such as the licensing of professionals and facilities or even direct public provision – are introduced to allocate resources and determine what kinds of care are provided. As an additional consequence, the poor functioning of markets creates opportunities for corruption, and the uncertainty inherent in selecting, monitoring, measuring and delivering healthcare services makes it difficult to detect and assign responsibility for abuses.[83]

But the degree of uncertainty is not identical for everyone in the health sector, leading to a second systemic feature, namely asymmetric information. Information is not shared equally among health sector actors and this has significant implications for a health system's efficiency and its vulnerability to corruption. Healthcare providers are better informed of the technical features of diagnosis and treatment than patients. Pharmaceutical companies know more about their products than the doctors who prescribe them, individuals have certain kinds of information about their health that are not available to medical care providers or insurers and providers and insurers may have better information about the health risks faced by certain categories of individuals than the individuals themselves.[84]

Finally, health systems are prone to corruption because of the large number of actors involved and the complexity of their multiple forms of interaction. These actors can be classified into five main categories:

- Government Regulators (health ministries, parliament, specialized commissions)
- Payers (social security institutions, government offices, private insurers)
- Providers (hospitals, doctors, pharmacists)
- Consumers (patients)
- Suppliers (medical equipment and pharmaceutical companies)

The presence of so many actors increases the difficulty of generating and analyzing information, promoting transparency and even identifying corruption when it occurs. It increases the number of opportunities for corruption; for example, funds can be diverted or misallocated at a ministry, state hospital or local clinic by individuals working as managers, procurement officers, health professionals, dispensers and clerk or patients. The involvement of so many actors multiplies the number and kinds of interest that might encourage corrupt behaviour.[85]

Ivan Illich in his brilliant work, *Medical Nemesis: The Expropriation of Health*, published in 1974, has exposed the acute crisis of the healthcare sector. The medical establishment has become a major threat to healthy living. Dependence on professional healthcare affects all social relations. In rich countries medical colonization has reached sickening proportions; poor countries are also following the line. Medicine is about to become a prime target for political action that aims at an invasion of industrial society.[86]

A professional healthcare system, which has grown beyond tolerable bounds, is sickening for three reasons:[87]

- It must produce clinical damages, which outweighs its potential benefits.
- It cannot but obscure political conditions, which render society unhealthy.
- It tends to expropriate the power of the individual to heal oneself and to shape his or her environment.

The medical or paramedical monopoly over hygienic methodology and technology is a glaring example of the political misuse of scientific achievements to strengthen industrial rather than personal growth. Illich thinks that such medicine is but a device to convince those who are sick and tired of the society, i.e., those who are ill, impotent and in need of technical repair.[88]

The changes in health status are generally equated with progress and are attributed to more or better medical care. In fact, there is no evidence of any direct relation between the changing form of the sickness and the so-called progress of medicine.

Illich correctly points out that the analysis of the disease trends shows that the environment is the primary determinant of the state of any population. Food, housing, working condition, neighbourhood cohesion, as well as cultural mechanisms play a decisive role in determining the health conditions of the individual.[89]

Following Illich, it is relevant to point out that the impact of medicine constitutes one of the most rapidly expanding epidemics of the present time. Medicines have always been potentially poisonous, but their unwanted side effects have increased with their effectiveness and widespread use.[90]

Changing healthcare culture has identified certain indications of the human body as diseases. Corporatization of healthcare has elevated the status of certain normal symptoms as 'disease' or 'sickness'. Pharmaceutical companies and hospitals are always in the process of detecting the abnormalities and syndromes and are keen to term them as a disease.

The changes in the social terrain of health and illness have 'medicalized' life to its fullest. It has created an atmosphere of sickness where the normal human beings are always under the threat of being ill. Medicalization leads to 'normal' human behaviour and experience being 're-badged' as a medical condition.[91]

One of the capabilities of medicine is to kill. Until recent times the negative effects of medicine remained inscribed within the register of medical ignorance. Medicine was killed through the doctor's ignorance or because medicine itself was ignorant. It was not a true science, but rather a rhapsody of an ill-founded, poorly established and undiversified set of knowledge. The harmfulness of medicine was judged in proportion to its non-scientificity.[92]

Cholesterol is an important component of blood. There has been an age-old idea that increasing cholesterol levels can cause cardiac arrest. However, cholesterol triglyceride acts as an important component of the human body. But over-popularizing the negative impact of cholesterol signified that its presence in blood can be harmful. The useful impacts of the medicines that are used to dilute the high cholesterol level are not yet properly discerned. But the side effects of these medicines can inevitably invite other diseases. Similar explanations can also be given in cases of osteoporosis, hypertension and diabetes.[93]

Medicines have thus become a new society fad. It is preconceived that there is a remedy for and against everything. The market is full of performance supporting pills and tonics claiming to strengthen the immunity defence system. The consumers of these small and multicoloured pills are not only old and ill but also an increasing number of healthy and young people who are becoming regular consumers of these drugs' disease mongering. Thus widening the boundaries of treatable illnesses in order to expand markets for those who sell and deliver treatments. The social construction of illness is being replaced by the corporate construction of disease.

Notes

1   M. Mackintosh and M. Koivusalo, eds, *Commercialisation of Health Care: Global and Local Dynamics and Policy Responses* (New York: Palgrave Macmillan, 2005), cited in Rama V. Baru, "Medical Industrial Complex: Trends in Corporatization of Health Services", in *Equity and Access: Health Care Studies in India*, ed. Purendra Prasad and Amar Jessani (New Delhi: OUP, 2018), 75 (Hereafter cited as Baru, "Medical Industrial Complex").
2   W.D. White, "The "Corporatization" of US Hospitals: What can We Learn from the Nineteenth Century Industrial Experience?" *International Journal of Health Services* 20, no. 1 (1990): 85–113.
3   A.S. Relman, "The New Medical Industrial Complex", *The New England Journal of Medicine* 303, no. 17 (1980): 963–70 and P. Starr, *The Social Transformation of American Medicine* (New York: Basic Books, 1982), cited in Baru, "Medical Industrial Complex", 75–76.
4   P. Bose, "India Presents Challenging Paradigms, Opportunities: Terri Bresenham". Interview with President and CEO, GE Healthcare India, *Business Standard*, 26 March 2012, cited in Indira Chakravarthi, "The Emerging 'Health Care Industry' in India: A Public Health Perspective", *Social Change* 43, no. 2 (2013): 165–76 (Hereafter cited as Chakravarthi, "Healthcare Industry").
5   FICCI (2008). Fostering Quality Healthcare for all. FICCI HEAL 2008, Federation of Indian Chambers of Commerce and Industry Health Services Division, New Delhi, cited in Chakravarthi, "Healthcare Industry".
6   Confederation of Indian Industry (CII) (2011). Addressing the unfinished agenda: Universal healthcare, cited in Chakravarthi, "Healthcare Industry".
7   http://www.article alley.com_882070_15.html Accessed on 14.06.2010.
8   Indira Chakravarthi, "Corporate Presence in the Health Care Sector in India", *Social Medicine* 5, no. 4 (December 2010) (www.socialmedicine.info). Accessed on 07.02.2021 (Hereafter cited as Chakravarthy, "Corporate Presence in Health Care Sector").
9   B. Levebre, "The Hospital Chains in India: The Coming of Age?" Published by Centre Asie Ifri (2010) cited in Baru, "Medical Industrial Complex", 83, Jeffery. Also see Chakravarthi, "Healthcare Industry".
10 Roger Jeffery, "Commercialisation in Health Service", in *Global Health Governance and Commercialisation of Public Health in India: Actors, Institutions and Dialectics of Global and Local,* ed. Anuj Kapilashrami and Rama V. Baru (UK: Routledge, 2019), 93.
11 S. Hodges, "Hospital Chains in India: Healthcare Myths and Their Making in Contemporary India", *Indian Journal of Medical Ethics* 10, no. 4 (2010): 242–49, cited in Baru, "Medical Industrial Complex", 81.
12 Ibid., 81.
13 Chakravarthy, "Corporate Presence in Health Care Sector", 194.
14 Ibid., 195.
15 https://www.fortishealthcare.com/ Accessed on 10.1.2022.
16 Chakravarthy, "Corporate Presence in Health Care Sector", 194.
17 Ibid.
18 https://www.livemint.com/Companies/1hab58fTdM4ULjzA3EWAyN/Fortis -completes-acquisition-of-Wockhardt-hospitals.html Accessed 10.01.2022.

19 Jeffery, "Commercialisation in Health Service", 93. Also see Chakravarthi, "Corporate Presence in Health Care Sector".
20 Chakravarthi, "Healthcare Industry", 168.
21 Chakravarthi, "Corporate Presence in Health Care Sector", 194.
22 Ibid.
23 Hooda, "Health Systems in Transition". Also see S. Sehgal and S. Hooda, "Emerging Role of Private Sector in Indian Health Care Delivery Market: Trends, Pattern and Implications", *Intern Report* (New Delhi: Institute for Studies in Industrial Development (ISID), 2015).
24 https://doi.org/10.1101/2020.06.16.20132787 Accessed on 14.09.2020.
25 Government of India, "*The Key Indicators on Health and Morbidity Survey, Round Number 71, 2014*", National Sample Survey Office (NSSO), Ministry of Statistics and Programme Implementation, Government of India (2014).
26 Shailender Kumar Hooda, "Foreign Investment in Hospital Sector In India: Trends, Pattern and Issues", *Working Paper 181*, April (2015) (New Delhi: Institute for Studies in Industrial Development). (Hereafter cited as Hooda, "Foreign Investment in Hospital Sector").
27 Pushpa Sharma and Chandan Sapkota. "Liberalising Health Services under the SAARC Agreement on Trade in Services (SATIS): Implications for Nepal". Report submitted to Centre for Policy Dialogue, Dhaka, Bangladesh, January 2011. https://www.academia.edu/25336788/liberalizing_health_services_under_the_SAARC_Agreement _on_Trade_in_Services_SATIS_Implications_for_Nepal Accessed on 21.06.2022.
28 Ibid.
29 Ibid.
30 Hooda, "Foreign Investment in Hospital Sector".
31 Investment Opportunities in India's Health Care Sector, Niti Ayog, March 2021.
32 www.ibef.org Accessed on 03.01.2022. Also see medical device imports.html Accessed on 3.12.2021.
33 Jeffery, "Commercialisation of Health Services", 85.
34 R. Ilaiyarani, *A Study on Role of Foreign Direct Investment in Healthcare Sector in India*. Synopsis submitted to Madurai Kamaraj University for the award of the Degree of Doctor of Philosophy in Business Administration (2019).
35 For more details see Jeffery, "Commercialisation of Health Services".
36 Jeffery, "Commercialisation of Health Services", 91.
37 Medical Device Industry in India, "The Evolving Opportunities, Landscape and Challenges", skpgroup.com, September 2017.
38 For more details, see the unpublished Phd thesis, titled "Health Care in Crisis: The Changing Pattern of Private Health Care in Post-Independence Kolkata". Available at http://hdl.handle.net/10603/176075.
39 See Chakravarthi, "Corporate Presence in Health Care Sector".
40 *Health on the March* (2016–2018).
41 *World Development Report: Investing in Health* (New York: OUP, 1993).
42 Ibid.
43 A. Banerji, A. Deaton, and E. Duflo, in the article "Health Care Delivery in Rural Rajasthan", *Ecnomic and Political Weekly* XXXIX, no. 9 (28 February 2004), mentioned that people spent substantially on healthcare largely provided by unqualified persons in the private sector where services were even worse. Yet over the 1990s, as India embarked upon its structural adjustment programme, state spending on health declined. Baru is of the opinion that the decline in public investments matched with growing subsidies to the private sector in healthcare in a variety of ways. S. Nandaraj in 'Private Health Sector in India' pointed out that in India, contracting had been initiated under the blindness programme and the AIDS control programme and franchising arrangements had been set up with private providers under the Revised National Tuberculosis Control Programme (RNTCP). Nandraj also mentioned the transfer of

ownership of a public care hospital in Mumbai as part of a state health system project funded by the World Bank. The Mumbai municipal corporation had taken a policy decision to hand over many of its peripheral hospitals to the private sector. In a controversial move, a peripheral hospital was also handed over to a private medical college that did not have the necessary clinical facilities; the Medical Council of India had not recognized the medical college concerned. Other cities, such as Ahmedabad, have handed over facilities to NGOs. However, the role of NGOs in supporting the public healthcare sector is also questionable. Duggal et al. (1986), Baru (1999) and Visaria (2002) have pointed out that in better off states, the performance of the NGOs are remarkably good.

Debashish Dutta, "Privatisation of Health: A Letter from West Bengal", http://ccih09.pbworks.com/f/a09roy+gaurab+(2).pdf Accessed on 13.12.2009.

Ajkaal (Bengali daily), 1 August 1995.

Seventeenth Report of the Standing Committee on Health and Family Welfare, 1999–2000, Twelfth Legislative Assembly, Report on Pre-Voting Budget Scrutiny (2000–2001), West Bengal Legislative Assembly Secretariate.

Ibid.

Economic Review 1998–99, Government of West Bengal.

44 *Economic Review* 1999–2000, Government of West Bengal.
45 *Economic Review* 2000–01, Government of West Bengal.
46 *Economic Review* 2001–02.
47 *Economic Review* 2002–03.
48 *Economic Review* 2003–04.
49 Ibid.
50 Ibid.
51 Ibid.
52 *Economic Review* 2005–06.
53 Ibid. Read Timir Kanti Das, *Monozyme Kit Kelenkari: Janaswasthyer Prati Sarkari Abahela, Udasinata o Simahin Durnitir ek Kalankajanak Adhyay* (Monozyme Kit Scam: An Episode of the State's Indifference, Negligence and Corruption towards Public Health), *Swasthya Bikshan*, Kolkata: Medical Service Centre, 12th year 2nd issue (January 2007); Priyanka Chatterji, *Daktari Sikhshar Banijyikaran: Sikshay Banijyikaraner ek Natun Adhyaye Paschimbanga* (Commercialization of Medical Education: A New Phase of Commercialization of Education in West Bengal), *People's Health*, Kolkata (November 2008).
54 Ibid.; Dutta, "Privatisation of Health: A Letter from West Bengal".
55 Ibid.; Das, "Monozyme Kit*Kelenkari*".
56 Ibid.; Dutta, "Privatisation of Health: A Letter from West Bengal".
57 Ibid. See Sabyasachi Mitra, *"Kemon Achho? Pashchimbanger Gramin Swasthya Byabasthya"* (How are You? Rural Healthcare in West Bengal), *Ekhan Bishambad* (March 2008); Asish Kumar Ghosh, *"Primary Health Centregulo Bartamane je Abasthay"* (Present Condition of the Primary Health Centres), *People's Health*, Kolkata (November 2008), and Indira Chakravarthy, "Public Health Privatization in Bengal", http://sanhati.com/front-page/857 Accessed on 6.6.2010.
58 Ibid.
59 Ibid.
60 Ibid.
61 Read Timir Kanti Das, *"Monozyme Kit Kelenkari"*; Priyanka Chatterji, *"Daktari SikhsharBanijyikaran"*. Also see Sabyasachi Mitra, *"Kemon Achho?"*; Asish Kumar Ghosh, *"Primary Health Centregulo Bartamane je Abasthay"* and Indira Chakravarthy, "Public Health Privatization in Bengal".
62 Bengal Global Business Summit 2017, *West Bengal, State Rides the Growth*. Also see the website of National Urban Health Missions.
63 *Health on the March* (2016–2018).

64 Kaveri Gill, "The Commodification of India's Health Care Services: Public Interests, Policy, and Costly Choices", in *Healers or Predators: Healthcare Corruption in India*, ed. Samiran Nundy and Sanjay Nagral (New Delhi: OUP, 2018), 66 (Hereafter cited as Nundy and Nagral, "Healers or Predators").

65 Mukhopadhaya, "Universal Health Coverage", 187–89.

66 Ritu Priya and Prachinkumar Ghodajkar, "The Structural Basis of Corruption in Healthcare in India", in *Healers or Pradators*, ed. Nundy and Nagral, 22–23 (Hereafter cited as Priya and Ghojkar, "The Srtuctural Basis of Corruption").

67 Ibid., 22.

68 Priya and Ghojkar, "The Srtuctural Basis of Corruption", 23.

69 N.H. Antia, "Missue of Medicine", in *Market Medicine and Malpractice*, ed. Amar Jesani, P.C. Singhi, and Padma Prakash (Mumbai: Centre for Enquiry into Health and Allied Themes (CEHAT) and Society for Public Health Awareness and Action (SPHAA), 1997), 9 (Hereafter cited as Antia, "Misuse of Medicine").

70 Interview with Dr N.C. Das on 10.08.2007.

71 Antia, "Misuse of Medicine", 9.

72 Priya and Ghojkar, "The Srtuctural Basis of Corruption", 23.

73 Ibid., 23.

74 Antia, "Misuse of Medicine", 11.

75 Sumit Ray, "Hospital Practices and Healthcare Corruption", in *Healers or Predators*, ed. Nundy and Nagral, 156–59.

76 For more details on negligence and malpractice see the unpublished Phd thesis, titled "Health Care in Crisis: The Changing Pattern of Private Health Care in Post-Independence Kolkata". Available at http://hdl.handle.net/10603/176075. Also see Kunal Saha, "My Battle with Medical Negligence" and Farokh Erach Udwadia "What Should We Do?", in *Healers or Predators*, ed. Nundy and Nagral, 519–32.

77 Ivan Iliich, *Medical Nemesis: The Expropriation of Health* (London: Calder and Boyars, 1974), 24 (Hereafter cited as Illich, *Medical Nemesis*).

78 L. Corey, M. Epsteinand, and S. Saltman, "Society for Health: Dilemma", in *Medicine in a Changing Society*, ed. L. Corey, M. Epstein, and S. Saltman (St Louis: The C.V. Mosby Company, 1977), 3.

79 Ibid., 3.

80 Ibid., 4.

81 William D. Savedoff and Karen Hussmann, "The Causes of Corruption in the Health Sector: A Focus on Health Care Systems", in *Global Corruption Report 2006* (London: Pluto, 2006), 4.

82 Kenneth J. Arrow, "Uncertainty and the Welfare Economics of Medical Care", *American Economic Review* 53 (1963), in William D. Savedoff and Karen Hussmann, "The Causes of Corruption in the Health Sector", 5.

83 Ibid., 5.

84 Ibid., 6.

85 Ibid.

86 Illich, *Medical Nemesis*, 11.

87 Ibid., 11.

88 Ibid.

89 Ibid.

90 Ibid., 17–22.

91 Irving Zola, "Medicine as an Institution of Social Control", *The Sociological Review* 20 (1972): 487–504, cited in Arunima Sarvdeep Kohli, "Medicalization: A Growing Menace", *Delhi Psychiatry Journal* 15, no. 2 (October 2012), 255. Hereafter cited as Kohli, "Medicalization: A Growing Menace".

92 Ibid. For more details on Medicalistion read Ray Moynihan, Iona Heath, and David Henry, "Selling Sickness: The Pharmaceutical Industry and Disease Mongering", *British Medical Journal* 324; Michael Foucault, "The Crisis of Medicine or the Crisis

of Antimedicine?", English translation by Edgar C. Knowlton Jr., William J. King and Clare O'Farrell in *Foucault Studies* no. 1 (2004): 5–19.
93 Nabendu Bhattacharya, *"Oshudh Bechte Ashukh Gachhao"* (Promote diseases to sell medicines), *People's Health*, May 2009, 13. Also read Amrita Bagchi, "Medicalisation' of Diseases: A Crisis in the Domain of Social Health", *Science and Culture* 86, no. 11–12 (2020).

References

Ajkaal (Bengali daily), 1 August 1995.
Bagchi, Amrita. *Health Care in Crisis: The Changing Pattern of Private Health Care in Post-Independence Kolkata.* Unpublished Phd thesis. http://hdl.handle.net/10603/176075.
Bagchi, Amrita. "Medicalisation' of Diseases: A Crisis in the Domain of Social Health". *Science and Culture* 86, no. 11–12 (2020): 357–362.
Banerji, A., A. Deaton, and E. Duflo. "Health Care Delivery in Rural Rajasthan". *Ecnomic and Political Weekly* XXXIX, no. 9 (2004): 944–949.
Bhattacharya, Nabendu. "Oshudh Bechte Ashukh Gachhao" (Promote diseases to sell medicines). *People's Health*, May 2009.
Chakravarthi, Indira. "Corporate Presence in the Health Care Sector in India". *Social Medicine* 5, no. 4 (2010) (www.socialmedicine.info).
Chakravarthi, Indira. "Public Health Privatization in Bengal". http://sanhati.com/front -page/857, 2007.
Chakravarthi, Indira. "The Emerging 'Health Care Industry in India': A Public Health Perspective". *Social Change* 43, no. 2 (2013): 165–176.
Chatterji, Priyanka. "Daktari Sikhshar Banijyikaran: Sikshay Banijyikaraner ek Natun Adhyaye Paschimbanga" (Commercialization of Medical Education: A New Phase of Commercialization of Education in West Bengal). Kolkata: People's Health, November 2008.
Corey, L., M. Epstein, and S. Saltman. *Medicine in a Changing Society.* Saint Locus: The C V Mosvy Company, 1977.
Das, Timir Kanti. "Monozyme Kit Kelenkari: Janaswasthyer Prati Sarkari Abahela, Udasinata o Simahin Durnitir ek Kalankajanak Adhyay" (Monozyme Kit Scam: An Episode of the State's Indifference, Negligence and Corruption towards Public Health). *Swasthya Bikshan.* Kolkata: Medical Service Centre, January 2007.
Dutta, Debashish. "Privatisation of Health: A Letter from West Bengal". http://ccih09 .pbworks.com/f/a09roy+gaurab+(2).pdf, 2009.
Foucault, Michael. "'The Crisis of Medicine or the Crisis of Antimedicine?'" *Foucault Studies* 1 (2004): 5–19. Translated by Edgar C. Knowlton, Jr., William J. King, and Clare O'Farrell.
Ghosh, Asish Kumar. "Primary Health Centregulo Bartamane je Abasthay" (Present Condition of the Primary Health Centres). Kolkata: People's Health, November 2008.
Government of India. "The Key Indicators on Health and Morbidity Survey, Round Number 71, 2014". National Sample Survey Office (NSSO), Ministry of Statistics and Programme Implementation, Government of India (2014).
Government of West Bengal, Directorate of Health Services. State Bureau of Health Intelligence, *Health on the March (2016–2018)*, 2004.
Government of West Bengal. *Economic Review.* Kolkata: Department of Planning and Statistics, Government of West Bengal (1998–2004).
Government of West Bengal. *West Bengal Human Development Report 2004.* Kolkata: Development and Planning Department, 2004.

Hooda, Shailendra. "Health System in Transition in India: Journey from State Provisioning to Privatization". *World Review of Political Economy* 11, no. 4 (Winter 2020): 63–84.

https://economictimes.indiatimes.com/industry/healthcare/biotech/healthcare/india-imports-80-of-its-requirement-of-medical-devices-mos-ashwini-choubey/articleshow/80885094.cms.

http://www.article alley.com_882070_15.html.

https://doi.org/10.1101/2020.06.16.20132787.

https://www.fortishealthcare.com.

https://www.livemint.com/Companies/1hab58fTdM4ULjzA3EWAyN/Fortis-completes-acquisition-of-Wockhardt-hospitals.html.

Ilaiyarani, R. "A Study on Role of Foreign Direct Investment in Healthcare Sector in India". Synopsis submitted to Madurai Kamaraj University for the award of the Degree of Doctor of Philosophy in Business Administration (2019).

Illich, Ivan. *Medical Nemesis: The Expropriation of Health.* London: Calder and Boyars, 1974.

Interview with Dr, N.C. Das on 10.08.2007, Kolkata.

Kapilashrami, Anuj, and Rama V. Baru, eds. *Global Health Governance and Commercialisation of Public Health in India: Actors, Institutions and Dialectics of Global and Local.* London and New York: Routledge, 2019.

Kohli, Arunima Sarvdeep. "Medicalization: A Growing Menace". *Delhi Psychiatry Journal* 15, no. 2 (October 2012): 255–259.

Medical Device Industry in India. "The Evolving Opportunities, Landscape and Challenges". September 2017. skpgroup.com.

Mitra, Sabyasachi. "Kemon Achho? Pashchimbanger Gramin Swasthya Byabasthya" (How are you? Rural healthcare in West Bengal). *Ekhan Bishambad,* March 2008.

Moynihan, Ray, Iona Heath, and David Henry. "Selling Sickness: The Pharmaceutical Industry and Disease Mongering". *British Medical Journal* 324 (2002): 886–891.

Nundy, Samiran, and Sanjay Nagral, eds. *Healers or Predators: Healthcare Corruption in India.* New Delhi: OUP, 2018.

Prasad, Purendra, and Amar Jessani, eds. *Equity and Access: Health Care Studies in India.* New Delhi: OUP, 2018.

Savedoff, William D., and K. Hussmann. *Global Corruption Report 2006.* London: Pluto, 2006.

Sehgal, S., and S. Hooda. "Emerging Role of Private Sector in Indian Health Care Delivery Market: Trends, Pattern and Implications". *Intern Report.* New Delhi: Institute for Studies in Industrial Development (ISID), 2015.

Sharma, Pushpa, and Chandan Sapkota. "Liberalising Health Services under the SAARC Agreement on Trade in Services (SATIS): Implications for Nepal". Report submitted to Centre for Policy Dialogue, Dhaka, Bangladesh, January 2011. https://www.academia.edu/25336788/liberalizing_health_services_under_the_SAARC_Agreement_on_Trade_in_Services_SATIS_Implications_for_Nepal. Accessed on 21.06.2022.

West Bengal Legislative Assembly Secretariat. "Seventeenth Report of the Standing Committee on Health and Family Welfare, 1999–2000". *Report on Pre-Voting Budget Scrutiny.* Twelvth Legislative Assembly (2000–2001).

White, W.D. "The "Corporatization" of US Hospitals: What can We Learn from the Nineteenth Century Industrial Experience?" *International Journal of Health Services* 20, no. 1 (1990): 85–113.

World Bank.*World Development Report: Investing in Health.* New York: OUP, 1993.

www.ibef.org.

Conclusion

'The State shall regard the raising of the level of nutrition and the standard of living of its people and the improvement of public health as among its primary duties'. This is reflected in the Article 47 of the Indian Constitution, as a pronouncement of one of the Directive Principles of State Policy.

In Article 38 (1) of the Constitution, India is referred to as a welfare state, and in Article 41, it urges the state to strive towards extending public assistance in 'cases of unemployment, old age, sickness and disablement, and in other cases of undeserved want'. The most significant for the present study is Article 14, which states that all citizens have an equal right to life. Indian Constitution never openly declares health as a human right.

After Independence, the newly emerged welfare state held itself duty bound to provide its citizens with adequate health services.

Promises of the welfare state were not kept. Thus, more than 70 years after the Indian Constitution was formally accepted, the Directive Principles of State Policy have largely remained empty promises.

But there is something that is of greater concern. The state had declared its duty towards its citizens. However, this duty and the promise thereof, in the minds of the nation's politicians and officialdom, was something that was a boon or bonus, not something which the citizen could claim as a right. It is to be noted in this regard that the Indian Constitution, while it pronounces public health as a state duty *does not* also categorically pronounce it a citizens' right. It was only decades after the Constitution was prepared that the Courts of India gradually argued that health was, for citizens of India, indeed a matter of justiciable right and viewing it as such was legitimate through a reading of Directive Principles combined with Article 21.[1]

However, notwithstanding legal and judicial recognition of the citizens' right to health, this right in actuality has no real recognition in the civic and political culture of India. No political battles have been fought on the issue of healthcare as a right. Thus, along with food, nutrition, access to safe water and education, healthcare still remains one of those crucial sectors that in reality remains beyond the actual rights' horizon of the Indian citizen. Therefore, despite judicial pronouncements and occasional administrative declarations, the majority of Indian citizens remain disempowered creatures in almost all things that matter in life.

DOI: 10.4324/9781003169475-7

So, on the one hand promises have not been kept, and on the other, rights in actuality do not exist. It is in this vacuum that private healthcare has entered as an income-generating and profit-making sector. In the rural areas, the need for healthcare is addressed largely through practitioners of traditional knowledge, paramedics and quacks of varying competence. Formally, recognized physicians and healthcare services are available mainly in the urban areas where more people can afford such services. But one must bear in mind that formally recognized private healthcare, in the form of nursing homes and private hospitals, remains beyond the means of the bulk of India's population.

The impact of liberalization on health and medicine in India explains how the priorities set by the World Bank link public health programmes to market forces in an intrinsic manner. The concept of public health means that the state takes all necessary matters of health of the population and this implies a huge amount of resources and capital needed for a whole nation. Public health services require huge capital and market mechanisms for its supplies. Public health enhances the consumption of medicine, but this did not mean that people are healthier.[2]Public health as the care of the sick has given way to some kind of consumption of designated packages. In this the state is the largest consumer of medicines and vaccines and gets inextricably bound with pharmaceutical companies.[3]

As advanced tertiary care becomes important at the cost of primary health, the medical equipment industry promotes the use of sophisticated technology made for the rich countries. This puts a low priority on curing 'technologically unchallenging but epidemiologically important infectious diseases. Research institutions in the Third World shift to topics of international significance but of little relevance to local health problems. (For instance, organ transplant or coronary bypass gets more attention than treating commonplace diseases like diarrhoea or fever.) This led to the strange situation where the invention of a drug calls for the invention of disease'.[4]

What logically follows is to incur profit from ill-health – the more people fall ill and the longer they remain ill, the larger the profit for the care provider. The fundamental inconsistency can also be illustrated by the simple demand and supply logic of the marketplace. It can be legitimately argued that the demand for healthcare will always be infinite, for there is really no limit that one can set on good health. Thus, the demand for healthcare will always outstrip supply, and hence, under 'free market' conditions, the cost of healthcare will always rise exponentially.[5]

The new notion of medicine does not aim at healing the disease. It is more an 'illness care'[6] rather than healthcare, which has the tendency not to cure the disease but to make the society more 'unhealthy'. Wellness of the population at large is not the desired goal because improving public health through preventive measures and strengthening primary healthcare services do not fall under the domain of the techno-centric approach of corporate medicine. So more a nation is sick, more profit can be incurred – is the principle of healthcare in the era of liberalization.

Susan Sontag in the study *Illness as Metaphor*[7] (1978) analyzes 'illness' as a significant metaphor as opposed to the idea of wellness. The study perceives disease as any state of discomfort, which she figuratively describes as 'the night-side of life, a more onerous citizenship. Everyone who is born holds dual citizen-ship, in the kingdom of the well and in the kingdom of the sick'. And there is no escape from this dual citizenship.

Following Ritu Priya, it is pertinent to point out that the Bhore Committee report was an excellent blueprint of technical public health. It was not purely medicalized in its paradigm for improving the population's health at large and focused on building a strong edifice of a public system of health services. It had no policy for the private sector in healthcare.[8]

It is against this backdrop that the history of corporatization of healthcare has been examined. But having accepted this basic backdrop, one can get along with understanding the birth, development and subsequent transformation of private healthcare as a subject that deserves a separate study. In the era of neoliberal-ism, the changes in healthcare from a service to a lucrative industry were indeed a long-drawn process. The beginnings were made in the early decades after Independence, something which we have examined to some extent in this work.

The early form of private in-house healthcare was the nursing homes that mushroomed in a metropolis of a newly independent country and served the well-to-do sections of the society in the decades of the 1950s, 1960s and 1970s. We have discussed the features of such nursing homes and the nature of entrepreneur-ship that led to their emergence.

The once-popular small nursing homes of Kolkata are largely being displaced by the rising big corporate 'five-star hotel'-like multi/super speciality hospitals, which are similar to *Branded Healthcare Mall*s. As a result, the section of the populace, which once used the small nursing homes, now finds the corporate hos-pitals as better places for treatment. Interestingly, the urban lower middle class with little solvency and health consciousness tried their best to treat their dear ones in these small nursing homes rather than in the overcrowded public hospi-tals. With the breakdown of the public healthcare infrastructure in the rural areas, relatively affluent patients from these regions also utilized these nursing homes. But the nursing homes no longer enjoyed their previous glory. With the rising of the chains of 'supermarkets' in the 'smart' and sprawling malls of a globalized metropolis, the old-fashioned, once-popular corner grocery shops of the localities have been marginalized. A similar fate has been experienced by the small nursing homes of Kolkata. *The big capital swallowed up the small capital.*

With the retreat of the welfare state, the ailments of the public hospitals became visible. The main deficiencies in public healthcare are seen to be negli-gence, administrative indifference, staff shortage, lack of hospital beds and unfair nexus with the local nursing homes. Added to this are the medical accidents and indiscretions that are seen to abound in the public hospitals and healthcare centres. Although some positive measures were taken in recent years, the government has given much stress to put huge amounts of public money into raising new hos-pital buildings. This could achieve no success except popularity, as no specific provision of specialists and supplies has been made and no proper responsibili-ties taken. Thus, instead of building healthcare infrastructure, a hollow top-heavy 'super structure' is erected as the bottom layer of the primary healthcare sector is grossly ill-equipped.

A somewhat different picture emerges in the private sector. Here the incidents of gross negligence are not absent. But what tends to dominate the scene in the private sector is *overemphasis on unnecessary investigation and medication, indiscriminate use of intensive care units, exorbitant charges of bed and other facilities* and *inhumanly commercial attitude of the medical personnel* in the hospitals.

With the proliferation of private nursing homes and hospitals healthcare is transformed into a mere purchasable commodity, similar to any other expensive product of the market, and that too a product whose quality remains deeply suspected. In such a situation, the quality of the treatment that an individual gets remains a function of his or her luck, social resources and purchasing power. And commercialization tends to do away with whatever values of medical commitment that resided in the concept of a sacred physician–patient relationship.

Corporatized healthcare has, besides the usual diagnostic and therapeutic interventions, created a novel entity known as the 'health package'. This amazing entity is based upon the recognition of each individual as a cluster of symptoms – describable as a set of numbers (ranging from, say, blood pressure to the value of C-reactive protein) or a set of curves or images. Moreover in an *Atmosphere of Sickness* it is the fear or anxiety of getting sick or ill that hegemonizes the mind rather than the healthy awareness or preventive measures necessary for ailments.

The atmosphere of the hospital, the knowledgeable and powerful physician and the application of techno-medicine do not allow the patient to reveal the truth to an unknown investigator. Lying in a bed surrounded by air jets, buttons and lights, invaded by tubes and wires ... transported to special laboratories and imaging facilities replete with blinking lights, strange sounds and unfamiliar personnel, it is little wonder that patients may lose their sense of reality. In fact, a patient gets afraid of revealing the realities. In actuality the application of modern, corporate medicine observes a patient as a separate case and not as a human body. The dehumanizing factors of modern techno-centric medicine threaten the patients from becoming further sick or ill within the medicalized atmosphere of the hospital. The fear of surrendering the body to the expertise of the physicians compels the patients and patient parties not to speak out even in adversities in the hospital.[9]

In an altogether different note Gawande,[10] a US-based surgeon, in the wonderful work titled *Complications*, mentioned that medicine had the larger uncertainties that even puzzled, at the same time amazed the physicians.

Armed with such packages and combining within a single campus a whole array of diagnostic and therapeutic facilities, the corporate hospital stands forth as a veritable industry. And in order to keep the industry running and spewing profit at desirable rates, the life of the patient, now a 'consumer', must be 'medicalized'.

The critiques of globalized and corporatized healthcare are justified, or at least mostly so. But they tend to miss a crucial point. Issuing a big 'NO' to corporatization of health services may be necessary, *but it is far from being sufficient*. One must remember that healthcare in India remained abysmally inadequate in all the decades prior to India's jumping on to the liberalization-privatization-globalizati on bandwagon. One must also remember that whether a few dozen more multispecialty hospitals are opened or not in metropolitan India remains of little concern to some 80 million who have to rush to the quack or paramedic or queue up outside the Primary Health Centre. Their problem is not the 'medicalization' of life but rather the absence of basic treatment. For them it is the question of winning the rights to these fundamentals.

Amartya Sen[11] pointed out that the dismal picture of India's healthcare is mainly due to the utter neglect of primary healthcare and the inability to understand the critically important role of universal healthcare. Primary healthcare also suffers from behavioural corruption. Secondly, he mentions that India has a hasty and premature reliance on the private health sector, which goes hand in hand with the neglect of public healthcare. Finally, he opines that the informational lacuna in general and the asymmetric information between the buyers and the sellers in the market for healthcare provide a rich arena for abuse and exploitation.

Finally, one aspect needs mentioning. Ensuring the health of the population under the Universal Health Coverage is not the solution to the problem of access to and equity in healthcare. The ideas of increasing public spending up to 2.5 per cent of the GDP an important prerequisite and eradication of out-of-pocket expenditure is extremely essential; there are certain important contradictions between the goal and the design, which need to be highlighted. Eradication of out-of-pocket expenditure is a narrow goal; it should rather be one of the key strategies to achieve 'health for all'. This distinction becomes important because the goal drives the strategy. 'Universal health coverage' and 'health for all' mean two entirely different things. 'Health for all' requires a progressive socialization of healthcare, gradual undoing of commoditization of healthcare and a primary healthcare approach integrated under the notion of social determinants. The 'universal coverage' merely means that a financing system is developed to cover a majority of people against out-of-pocket expenditure but provisioning is done essentially through the market.[12]

In this context we can argue that the neoliberal turn has eroded the concept of health as a 'public good'. India's governments must realize that healthcare is a public good and is the state's responsibility. Public health is a 'public good'; i.e., its benefits cannot be individually enjoyed or computed but have to be seen in the context of benefits that are enjoyed by the public. Thus, public health outcomes are shared, and their accumulation leads to better living conditions. It does not mechanically translate into visible economic determinants, viz., income levels or rates of economic growth. The current economic policies would rather view health as a private good that is accessed through the market.[13]

The Government of India recently launched the Ayushman Bharat programme, which has two components of Prime Minister Jan Aarogya Yojana (hospitalization cover for the bottom 45 per cent of the population) and the health and wellness centres to consolidate primary healthcare. The former has been initiated to support insurance and private health sectors, but the latter, which should form the foundation for the former has been ignored and no significant budget allocation has been made for it. State-sponsored health insurances in reality promote not only the large-scale utilization of hospital beds in the private sector for public purposes but also result in channelizing public funds to the private sector, contracting of the existing public healthcare sector and deepening of the crisis of getting proper treatment from the giant corporates of the health sector. On the other hand, the abolition of user fees and introduction of free services in government hospitals are partially a real story because free services are seldom available without 'paying' a section of the employees or their agents at every level.

Notes

1 See in this connection K. Mathiharan, "The Fundamental Right to Health Care", *Indian Journal of Medical Ethics* 11, no. 4 (October–December 2003), http://www.issuesi nmedicalethics.org/114hl123.html and the relevant sources cited therein. Accessed on 10.06.2010.
2 Sujatha, *Sociology of Medicine*, 234.
3 Ibid.
4 Ibid.
5 See *Globalisation and Health* (Delhi: National Coordination Committee, Jan Swasthya Abhiyan, 2006).
6 See Bishan Basu, *Kine Ana Swasthya: Bajar-Punji-Munafa arApni* (Buying Health: Market-Capital-Profit and You) (Kolkata: Dhansiri, 2020).
7 Susan Sontag, *Illness as Metaphor* (New York: Farrar, Straus and Giroux, 1978).
8 Priya, "State, Community, and Primary Health Care", 42.
9 See Jayanta Bhattacharya, *Bio Medicine theke najardari medicine* (From Bio Medicine to Surveillance Medicine) (Kolkata, 2008). Here we can also refer to the Ullysses Syndrome where the patient undergoes a series of investigations under the physician for a longer period of time but cannot come to any detection. By the time the patient gets already cured but loses mental and physical strength and gets converted to a 'sick' individual. For more details see Sthabir Dasgupta, *Swasthya Niye Badbisongbad* (Debates over Health Issues) (Kolkata: Ananda Publishers, 2020).
10 Atul Gawande, *Complications* (Gurgaon: Penguin, 2002).
11 Amartya Sen, "Foreword", in Nundy and Nagral, *Healers or Pradators*, viii–xiii.
12 Mukhopadhyay, "Universal Health Coverage", 178–79.
13 See Jan Swasthya Abhiyan, *Globalisation and Health*; Ravi Duggal, "Making Healthcare a Public Good", *Economic and Political Weekly* 53, no. 14 (7 April 2018).

References

Basu, Bishan. *Kine Ana Swasthya: Bajar-Punji-Munafa ar Apni* (*Buying health: Market-capital-profit and you*). Kolkata: Dhansiri, 2020.
Bhattacharya, Jayanta. *Bio Medicine theke najardari Medicine*. Kolkata: Ababhash. 2008.
Dasgupta, Sthabir. *Swasthya Niye Badbisongbad* (*Debates over health issues*). Kolkata: Ananda Publishers, 2020.
Duggal, Ravi. "Making Healthcare a Public Good". *Economic and Political Weekly* 53, no. 14 (2018). 9.
Gawande, Atul. *Complications*. Gurgaon: Penguin, 2002.
Jan Swasthya Abhiyan. *Globalisation and Health*. Delhi: National Coordination Committee, 2006.

Mathiharan, K. "The Fundamental Right to Health Care". *Indian Journal of Medical Ethics* 11, no. 4 (October–December 2003), http://www.issuesinmedicalethics.org/114hl123 .html.

Mukhopadhyay, Indranil. "Universal Health Coverage: The New Face of Neoliberalism". *Social Change* 43 (2013). 177–190.

Nundy, Samiran, and Sanjay Nagral, eds. *Healers or Predators: Healthcare Corruption in India.* New Delhi: OUP, 2018.

Prasad, Purendra, and Jessani Amar, eds. *Equity and Access: Health Care Studies in India.* New Delhi: OUP, 2018.

Rao, K. Sujatha. *Do We Care? India's Health System.* New Delhi: OUP, 2020.

Sontag, Susan. *Illness as Metaphor.* New York: Farrar, Straus and Giroux, 1978.

Index